What Do I Say?

What Do I Say?

Communicating Intended or Unanticipated Outcomes in Obstetrics

James R. Woods Jr.
Fay A. Rozovsky

Foreword by David S. Guzick

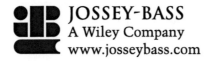

JOSSEY-BASS
A Wiley Company
www.josseybass.com

Published by Jossey-Bass
A Wiley Imprint
989 Market Street, San Francisco, CA 94103-1741 www.josseybass.com

This publication is designed to provide accurate and authoritative information in regard to the subject matter covered. It is sold with the understanding that the publisher is not engaged in rendering professional services. If professional advice or other expert assistance is required, the services of a competent professional person should be sought.

Jossey-Bass books and products are available through most bookstores. To contact Jossey-Bass directly call our Customer Care Department within the U.S. at 800-956-7739, outside the U.S. at 317-572-3993 or fax 317-572-4002.

Jossey-Bass also publishes its books in a variety of electronic formats. Some content that appears in print may not be available in electronic books.

Library of Congress Cataloging-in-Publication Data

Woods Jr., James R., 1943-
     What do I say? : communicating intended or unanticipated outcomes in obstetrics / James R. Woods Jr., Fay A. Rozovsky.
        p. ; cm.
     Includes bibliographical references and index.
     ISBN 0-7879-6654-1 (alk. paper)
     1. Obstetrics. 2. Informed consent (Medical law) 3. Medical personnel and patient. 4. Patient education.
     [DNLM: 1. Pregnancy Outcome—psychology. 2. Informed Consent. 3. Physician-Patient Relations. 4. Truth Disclosure. WQ 240 W895w 2002] I. Title: Communicating intended or unanticipated outcomes in obstetrics. II. Rozovsky, F. A. (Fay Adrienne), 1950- III. Title.
     RG526 .W665 2002
     618.2—dc21   2002154039

HC Printing   10 9 8 7 6 5 4 3 2 1   FIRST EDITION

CONTENTS

FOREWORD

In the course of physician training, from medical school through residency, the focus is on the acquisition of scientific and clinical knowledge, as well as procedural educational skill. The outcome of a clinical intervention, however, depends on a great deal more than knowledge and skill; it hinges on the relationship between a physician and his or her patient, which in turn depends on the nature of the communication between the physician and patient.

Virtually all experienced physicians would agree with the assertion that doctor-patient communication plays a key role in clinical outcomes, alongside knowledge and skill. Yet little time is spent in our medical schools on doctor-patient communication. Even less time is spent on doctor-patient communication in residency and fellowship training or in postgraduate courses for practicing physicians. Having spent seven years as chairperson of the Department of Obstetrics and Gynecology at the University of Rochester, as well as twenty years as a practicing clinician, I can confidently state that effective doctor-patient communication at once improves patient outcomes and limits the risk of lawsuits when a bad outcome occurs.

Make no mistake: improved communication will not solve the developing crisis in medical professional liability. In some states, a single jury verdict exceeds the sum of all obstetric professional liability premiums for a year. Moreover, there is a fundamental conflict between the incentives underlying our tort system and the reality of a baseline rate of adverse obstetric outcomes between 5 and 10 percent, independent of obstetric practice. However, physicians can markedly reduce their exposure to malpractice claims and, more important, establish better outcomes for their patients on a day-to-day basis by improving their communication with patients. It is for this reason that this book by James Woods and Fay Rozovsky is so welcome and timely.

Woods, a senior specialist in maternal fetal medicine (and my successor as chairperson of the Department of Obstetrics and Gynecology at the University of Rochester), and Rozovsky, an attorney who specializes in health care risk management, have teamed up to produce a unique book on strategies for communication in obstetrics. Suppose a bad outcome occurs in an obstetric patient. What are the perspectives of the patient, the insurer, and government? What are the legal issues around evidentiary protection and disclosure? Roszovsky considers these issues in an insightful and scholarly manner and also provides a comprehensive discussion of informed consent as a process underlying the doctor-patient relationship. Woods then relates a number of case-based scenarios on a variety of themes related to communication in obstetrics. Although these are hypothetical case studies, they represent a patchwork of clinical episodes that have come to Woods's attention during the course of his career in obstetrics. He then provides very specific, concrete advice on how to communicate effectively to patients and their families when adverse events occur.

From my personal experience of having observed Dr. Woods at work over many years, I can attest that he has often taken a clinical situation on an obstetrics service that has the potential to develop into a medical legal crisis and, through effective communication, transformed it into an expression of appreciation rather than a notice of legal action.

This is truly a unique book in the field of medicine, and it has implications far beyond obstetrics. The dual principles of informed consent as a fundamental process underlying the doctor-patient relationship and of forthright communication with patients and their families as the bedrock of the doctor-patient relationship will serve clinicians and their patients well in all branches of medical practice.

David S. Guzick, M.D., Ph.D.

PREFACE

Initiating a conversation with an obstetric patient to provide informed consent by explaining risks of an intended procedure or process is a health care challenge. To initiate that conversation when unanticipated adverse events occur is the nightmare feared by all health care providers.

Our role as obstetric care providers is to educate our patient and her family members so thoroughly about the care she is receiving and the risks or alternatives to that care that she becomes an equal participant in the final decisions regarding her body. Her family then becomes the knowledgeable support system for her selection of choices.

But what happens when an unanticipated adverse outcome occurs in obstetrics? Like leaves in a stream, the patient momentarily loses complete control over her life. She and her family are catapulted into a sea of grief, emptiness, confusion, indecision, and even anger. Her anchor in this emotional sea should be her care provider. For the care provider, however, thoughts such as, "Did I miss something?" or "Could I have done more to prevent this?" obscure what should be the intended role: to express compassion, educate, and provide continuity of care, even if the outcome was not as expected.

The ideas in this book are not uniquely ours. They reflect the many conversations and counseling sessions that we have observed or in which we have participated. It is often said that one voice cannot make a difference. That is not so. Each patient and/or her partner have taught us something new as she or he has shared experiences. Collectively, these voices are a road map toward communicating with those who seek our care. Their stories and the coping skills that they bring to this process illustrate the strength of the human spirit.

ACKNOWLEDGMENTS

We thank the following individuals at the University of Rochester for their help in the preparation of this book: Eva K. Pressman, associate professor of obstetrics and gynecology and director of obstetrics and maternal-fetal medicine; Jane Greenlaw, director of the Division of the Medical Humanities and codirector of the Program in Clinical Ethics; Deborah S. Phillips, clinical chief for obstetrics and gynecology nursing; and Mary Fisher, assistant to the chair of obstetrics and gynecology.

James R. Woods, Jr.
Fay A. Rozovsky

THE AUTHORS

James R. Woods Jr. is the Henry A. Thiede Professor and chair of the Department of Obstetrics and Gynecology at the University of Rochester School of Medicine, Rochester, New York. He completed medical school at Bowman Gray School of Medicine, his residency in obstetrics and gynecology at Tripler Army Medical Center in Hawaii, and his perinatal fellowship at the UCLA School of Medicine. Woods has authored and coauthored over 140 articles on maternal-fetal medicine, maternal drug addiction, complications of pregnancy, and clinical research. His book publications include *Pregnancy Loss, Medical Therapeutics and Practical Considerations,* and *Loss in Pregnancy or in the Newborn Period.* He has served as a regular member of a National Institutes of Health Study Section (NIDA) and as guest editor for *Clinical Obstetrics and Gynecology* and *Obstetrics and Gynecology Clinics of North America.* In 1996, an endowed chair honoring him was established at the University of Rochester. He has been named in *Best Doctors in America* for many years. Woods has lectured extensively on loss and grief in the medical setting. He has pioneered strategies for transforming some of the most challenging clinical interactions with patients after adverse outcomes into extraordinary opportunities for compassionate connection between clinicians and their patients and family members.

Fay A. Rozovsky is Senior Vice President of the Healthcare Practice of Marsh USA Inc. and has over twenty years of experience as a health care risk management consultant and attorney. She has lectured extensively and authored or coauthored over five hundred articles and several books, including *Consent to Treatment: A Practical Guide* (3rd ed.) and *Managing the Risks and Strategies for Physicians in Managed Care.* A graduate of Providence College, Rozovsky received a J.D. from Boston College Law School and an M.P.H. from the Harvard School of Public Health. She is an affiliate associate professor in the Department of Legal Medicine at the Medical College of Virginia and a Distinguished Fellow and past president of the American Society for Healthcare Risk Management. Currently, she is the vice chair of the Professional Technical Advisory Committee for Hospitals of the Joint Commission on Accreditation of Healthcare Organizations.

What Do I Say?

CHAPTER 1

The Legal Context for Disclosing Bad News

The health care industry is like a ship being tossed by high waves in the middle of a severe storm. It is being buffeted by angry and often distrusting patients, regulators, and legislators calling for rigorous scrutiny and payers demanding evidence-based quality care. At the same time, litigation-minded lawyers have fomented a wave of malpractice. The result has been a contracting of insurance carriers willing to write health professional liability insurance coverage. Those who are left in the field are demanding very expensive premiums for less coverage than was available only a few years ago. In the malpractice cases that go to trial, juries are sending a signal that the health care industry must transform itself into a quality-driven, accountable endeavor or be prepared to take the consequences in large damage awards.

To understand why there is so much emphasis on patient communication in the health care field, it is important to reflect on the drivers of this change: the change agents found in the government, accreditation, consumer, and payer sectors. Although many may not welcome this pressure for change, the result may be a health care system better prepared to partner with patients in the delivery of quality treatment and services.

THE FEDERAL PERSPECTIVE

In 1999, the Institute of Medicine (IOM) issued a landmark report that seemed to capture these shifting winds of dissatisfaction and distrust. In *To Err Is Human: Building a Safer Health System*, the IOM noted that the American health care industry kills an estimated forty-four thousand to ninety-eight thousand patients every year through medical error-related events.[1] The report pointed out that many of these deaths were preventable. Subsequently, a number of federal entities known as the Quality Interagency Coordination (QuIC) Task Force made their own recommendations in response to the IOM report. This QuIC report, *Doing What Counts for Patient Safety: Federal Actions to Reduce Medical Errors and Their Impact*, delineated one hundred action items for the federal government to take to rectify the situation.[2] In part, the government strategy focused on institutional accountability, leadership, and communication.

After the QuIC report, the Agency for Health Care Research and Quality (AHRQ; formerly known as the Agency for Health Care Policy and Research) took on a leadership role among federal authorities committed to patient safety. AHRQ has funded a variety of studies and research. One particular report, *Making Health Care Safer: A Critical Analysis of Patient Safety Practices*, reflects AHRQ's research commitment.[3] Prepared by the University of California at San Francisco (UCSF)–Standard Evidence-Based Practice Center (EPC), it focuses on evidence-based patient safety practices.

Working with the National Forum for Quality Measurement and Report, better known as the National Quality Forum (NQF), a partnership of private and public sector entities, the EPC developed a definition for a patient safety practice: "a type of process or structure whose application reduces the probability of adverse events resulting from exposure to the health care system across a range of diseases and procedures."[4] This definition encompasses communication skills and consent to treatment. Indeed, the report contained a discussion about informed consent and the need for research on the topic in conjunction with patient safety practices.

The Food and Drug Administration,[5] the Conditions of Participation for Hospitals in Medicare and Medicaid Patients Rights Standards,[6] and federally sponsored reports addressing the issue of patients rights[7] all point to the need for strong communication processes. Involving the patient in the decision-making process is viewed as a key ingredient to successful medical treatment.[8]

THE STATE GOVERNMENT PERSPECTIVE

At the state level, the move toward patient safety has been demonstrated by legislative initiatives geared toward reporting serious adverse events or patient deaths to databases in the belief that collecting such information will be useful in holding health care entities accountable for their performance.[9] As distinguished from voluntary reporting methodologies, the mandatory reporting procedures found in some states are at times linked to fines and penalties, and the format is tied to public disclosure.[10]

Some innovations have also occurred at the state level to facilitate reporting of adverse events without fear of disclosure of this information in medical malpractice litigation. The idea is to create an atmosphere conducive to the examination of adverse event information with a view to process improvement in patient safety. Examples of this approach include evidentiary use laws in Oklahoma,[11] Minnesota,[12] and Louisiana.[13] However, these laws are more the exception than the rule.

In addition, at the urging of the IOM in *To Err Is Human: Building a Safer Health System,* consideration is being given to a rethinking of health professional licensure at the state level.[14] The intent is to consider a variety of methodologies, including periodic relicensure.

The IOM report also emphasized the need for institutional accountability on the part of health care facilities. Indeed, *To Err Is Human: Building a Safer Health System* explored the idea of enterprise liability, that is, holding health care entities legally responsible for the errors and omissions of nonemployee health professionals who had been accorded staff privileges.[15] According to this concept, the health care entity could not avoid liability even when it contracted out delivery of health care services to physician groups for such departments as radiology or emergency medicine. Following the logic of this enterprise accountability theory, the hospital could be held negligent for a substandard consent to treatment on the part of a staff physician.

Thus far, only two states have clearly adopted the legal theory of enterprise liability.[16] In neither instance was consent the issue. Rather, it was the matter of substandard delivery of emergency treatment. However, at least one court has examined the idea of enterprise liability for negligent consent.[17] The point is that consent and the communication process underlying it may well be the basis for holding a hospital responsible for the negligence of a staff doctor. This type of liability exposure gives impetus to those who are trying to improve provider-patient communications and discussion of negative treatment outcomes.[18]

THE ACCREDITATION PERSPECTIVE

The Joint Commission on Accreditation of Healthcare Organizations (JCAHO) is the accrediting body for hospitals in the United States. In addition, it accredits nursing homes, integrated delivery systems, managed care organizations, and other health care organizations. The accreditation process is about quality of care, safe environments of care, and patient safety. It requires health care organizations to demonstrate compliance with standards developed for guiding health care services. Surveys are done to compare performance with the standards, and depending on the outcome, a health care entity may or may not receive a grade that is comparable to similarly situated facilities. Facilities that are in noncompliance will receive what are known as Type I or Type II findings, which require work to align the organization with the standards. In serious standards noncompliance situations, JCAHO may revoke or deny accreditation status.

Accreditation is a voluntary process. However, by becoming accredited, a hospital can host approved medical residency programs. Moreover, an accredited health care organization is automatically qualified to participate in Medicare and Medicaid. It need not seek separate approval from either the Centers for Medicare and Medicaid Services (CMS) or a state agency. Moreover, many health plans require JCAHO accreditation to be a participating provider for members, and many professional liability carriers look to JCAHO accreditation as a key indicator in deciding whether to offer insurance coverage.

At its best, the accreditation survey process is but a snapshot in time. In the interval between the previous survey and the subsequent evaluation, many things can happen that can result in a poor level of care or diminished patient safety. This fact was recognized in reports issued by the Government Accounting Office (GAO) and the Office of the Inspector General (OIG) of the U.S. Department of Health and Human Services.

Calling into question the value of the costly accreditation process, both the GAO and the OIG made several criticisms that went to the core of the JCAHO process.[19] JCAHO responded by revamping many aspects of the accreditation model. The reformation is ongoing to make the accreditation process more efficient, practical, and directed to delivery of high-quality, patient-safe care.

As a result of publication of *To Err Is Human,* JCAHO ramped up its efforts in patient safety.[20] Indeed, it is noteworthy that prior to publication of this IOM report, JCAHO had embarked on a course of reducing risk-prone processes through the use of root cause analysis for what it termed reviewable sentinel events. Borrowing a page from industry, JCAHO set out to have accredited facilities drill down into the systems failures that gave rise to patient injury or death. The vehicle for this effort was root cause analysis, which would pinpoint the common, latent, and special causes of iatrogenic illness or death.[21]

After the IOM report, JCAHO stepped up its activity, introducing a set of so-called patient safety standards designed to address a variety of systemic concerns that contribute to patient injury. Among the many patient safety standards is one that mandates a discussion of the outcomes of care with patients. JCAHO requires that patients, and when appropriate their families, receive information about the outcomes of care.[22] *Outcomes* here refers to both anticipated and unanticipated results, whether good or bad. However, JCAHO placed emphasis on the unanticipated outcomes of care, believing that doctors and other caregivers are reticent to share bad news with patients.

Many in the health care community interpreted the JCAHO requirement as compelling doctors and other health care professionals to make an admission of liability, although JCAHO adamantly denied this was the case. Others questioned how one could share bad outcome information with patients and their loved ones without leaving the implication of medical malpractice liability. The American Society for Healthcare Risk Management (ASHRM) issued a white paper on the subject that provided some perspectives on delivering such information without making an admission of culpability.[23] It has proved to be a good starting point for managing disclosure of unanticipated outcomes of care.[24] The ASHRM white paper emphasizes the need for frank and candid discussion of risks and benefits with patients prior to embarking on treatment. It views consent as laying the foundation for solid communications with patients and family members so that should unanticipated events occur, there is a preexisting relationship and framework for subsequent discussions.

JCAHO also has embarked on a new strategy to involve patients in their own care better. Termed "Speak Up: Help Prevent Errors in Your Care," this public relations strategy was designed to motivate patients to become more involved and informed participants as members of the health care team. According to JCAHO, the new concept is based on research demonstrating "that patients who take part in decisions about their health care are more likely to have better outcomes."[25] At the core of the initiative is the enhancement of professional-patient communications.

There is little doubt that the JCAHO's patients' safety standards are a key driver of change shaping the delivery of safe care to patients.

PRESIDENT'S ADVISORY COMMISSION ON CONSUMER PROTECTION AND QUALITY IN THE HEALTHCARE COMMUNITY

In 1999, a report was published on the findings and recommendations of the President's Advisory Commission on Consumer Protection and Quality in the Healthcare Industry.[26] Not only did it address accessibility and affordability of health care services, it stressed the needs to involve patients better in designing treatment plans and for patients to have sufficient communication with health care providers. Tying information to the quality of health care, the report reinforced the idea of a patient's right to information. As such, it became an important driver in the push for patient safety.

THE PAYER PERSPECTIVE

Payers have many interests in promoting quality-based health care. With so many employers paying ever-increasing premiums for health care coverage, there is an expectation that the money should be spent wisely in promoting wellness and curing illness. When employees complain that care is inadequate or shoddy or that they come away from a health care encounter injured, employers have reason to be concerned. Not only does this suggest that health care premiums are not being spent wisely, but employers may not be meeting their obligations under federally qualified health care plans. At the same time, employers worry about worker productivity if health care does more harm than good.

In January 2000, a group of the Fortune 500 from the Business Roundtable formed a coalition called "The Leapfrog Group" to respond to the situation.[27] With a mandate to alter the situation in terms of patient safety, Leapfrog has positioned itself to jump over government regulatory inroads and accreditation standards to effect change. In 2001, it published three standards for hospitals to meet: referrals to facilities that have a high volume of procedures, computerized order entry, and use of intensivists in intensive care units. The idea was that these three steps would start the health care industry down the road to effective change. In 2002, it completed a survey of hospital compliance with the standards. More standards are expected in future.

The payer is not going to remain silent. Increased health care costs, employee dissatisfaction, and perceived quality-of-care issues are driving the formation of so-called baby Leapfrogs, or state-based initiatives to compel change. Greater participation of employees in treatment planning is seen as a key point, especially with the results of benchmark studies designed to inform consumers about how well hospitals compare with one another in the delivery of care based on the Leapfrog standards.

THE CONSUMER PERSPECTIVE

The President's Advisory Commission Report is a reflection of the concerns articulated by consumers. Many are afraid to seek health care. They fear becoming another medical error statistic. They want more information, not less, about their health care. Many want to know about the treatment or outcome results of a surgeon who proposes to perform a surgical procedure. Others want information about hospital performance, medication error rates, and infection control statistics before seeking treatment at an acute care facility.[28] Web site–based information is becoming available on disciplinary activity surrounding physicians, data made available through the auspices of some state boards of medicine.[29] JCAHO publishes "Quality Check" data on hospital performance, information that is easily accessible over the Internet.[30]

The point is that consumers want to make informed choices about their health care. Knowing the "batting average" of a doctor or a hospital is important to consumers in deciding from whom to seek health care services. To consumer groups, making this information available to the public helps drive competition for the delivery of quality, patient-safe health care services.

THE INSURANCE INDUSTRY PERSPECTIVE

Beyond legislative, regulatory, accreditation, payer, and consumer-driven demands for greater disclosure of information, there are other key groups to consider. One group in particular is the medical malpractice or professional health care liability insurance carriers.

In many instances, insurance carriers have been seen as an impediment to disclosure of information about adverse outcomes of tests or treatment. It has been posited that physicians have been admonished by carriers *not to* reveal such information voluntarily lest it be seen as an admission of liability. Should physicians reject such direction from their insurance carriers, they may face the prospect of a so-called reservation of rights letter, in which the insured is told that coverage may not be available for making disclosures that compromise the ability to properly defend any claims arising out of the unanticipated or adverse outcome.

To be sure, the insurance industry may be sending mixed messages. Some insurers have taken a very public stance in encouraging their insured physicians to communicate with patients about unanticipated outcomes of care.[31]

Perhaps there is a plausible explanation for the apparent disagreement, perceived or real, among liability insurance carriers. Insurers do not want to set the stage for an antagonistic battle between a staff physician and a hospital, an approach that could easily backfire in the course of building a joint defense strategy. Furthermore, liability carriers do not want hospitals to be forced to choose between listening to a "say nothing" approach from an insurer, on the one hand, and, on the other, facing accreditation repercussions if they do not abide by the patient safety standard on disclosure of unanticipated outcomes of care.

The middle ground in each instance focuses on disclosure of information about outcomes of care without making admissions of liability. Such an approach is plausible and achievable if a factual account is presented without making statements that point the finger of culpability in the direction of a specific caregiver or health care organization. In drawing a distinction between disclosure of adverse outcome information and a statement steeped in blame or fault, some liability insurance carriers do not exhibit any difficulty with their insured physicians' meeting the expectation to reveal details about unanticipated treatment results.

RESEARCH ON DISCLOSURE OF ADVERSE OUTCOMES
Articles and study results have been published that suggest that in appropriate circumstances, disclosure of adverse outcomes may thwart rather than exacerbate the chance for litigation stemming from the event. In one

study, surveys mailed to 400 patients sought to obtain patients' reactions to three hypothetical scenarios involving medical error. Most of the 149 respondents wanted the doctor to disclose when a mistake occurred, with most wanting an acknowledgment that an error had taken place. Interestingly, the study showed that doctors were likely to be sued or be reported if they *did not* acknowledge that a mistake had occurred. As the study investigators indicated, based on the findings in this patient sample, the failure to report medical errors actually increases the risk of lawsuits and professional disciplinary sanctions.[32]

An obvious concern about disclosure is the financial cost of acknowledging that an error has occurred. If a physician or a health care organization adopts a disclosure policy, will such revelations increase the ultimate cost of a malpractice claim or settlement? One study done at the Veterans Administration (VA) Medical Center in Lexington, Kentucky, suggests that the costs may actually decrease. Since adopting a disclosure policy, the Lexington facility has found that it has brought its claims or settlements down to the lowest amount paid for such events among a group of VA hospitals.[33]

To be sure, such studies can be criticized as representing a very small sample. Also, in the case of the VA findings, physician-employees cannot be sued in their individual capacity, a key protective benefit from the Federal Torts Claims Act.[34] Nonetheless, the results point to an important finding: communicating with patients and sharing with them details about adverse events can diffuse a situation that might otherwise lead to onerous litigation, professional disciplinary actions, and regulatory entanglements. Furthermore, there is no guarantee that a person with a predisposition to sue will be placated by disclosure about an adverse event. What the discussion may do in such instances is trigger an early, just, and financially reasonable settlement. This may be a win for health care professionals and organizations alike that are increasingly burdened by either escalating premiums for medical malpractice and health facility liability insurance or limitations in coverage. At the very least, the timing, setting, and scope of disclosure of bad news merit further research.

PRACTICAL CONSIDERATIONS

Other groups have their own perspectives on why there is a problem today in the health care field. Among them are professional trade associations that represent the interests of hospitals, physicians, and nurses;[35] health care professional unions; group purchasing associations;[36] the plaintiffs' bar; and defense attorneys. There are also experts in the field of health care public policy who have their own views on the subject.[37]

There are also a number of practical considerations—for example:

- A perception that doctors must see many more patients and spend less time with them than in the past due to the financial constraints imposed on them by managed care organizations and health plans
- A perception that consent is a form, not a process
- An absence of communications training for health care professionals that sets them up for failure in terms of successfully completing an effective consent process
- A lack of communications training for health care professionals that makes them incapable of dealing with disclosure of unanticipated outcomes

Many of these considerations are easily dispelled. For example, as noted in Chapter Two, consent is *not* a piece of paper; rather, it is a communications process. Similarly, even if caregivers never received formal training on the proper methods for communicating information to patients, they can learn to do so through continuing-education programs. Moreover, with tools such as checklists, it is possible to curtail the amount of time perceived as being required to complete a successful consent process.

Anyone can put up hurdles to thwart change. The old paradigm of silence about bad outcomes has begun to fall by the wayside. In its place is a practical framework guided by cogent legal advice and proper training for those who must deliver the bad news.

THE LEGAL PROBLEM: EVIDENTIARY PROTECTION AND DISCLOSURE

By far, one of the most challenging issues is the matter of evidentiary protection in situations in which health care professionals must disclose information regarding adverse outcomes. Given the state of evidentiary laws, this is a very real concern.

In the United States, there is not a single consistent legislative, regulatory, or case law approach to the issue of evidentiary protection for the review of adverse events. In many instances, the results of such reviews, including root cause analysis, could be subject to legal discovery or admitted as evidence in a professional liability claim. This is seen as having a chilling effect on health care professionals' taking part in such activities even though the purpose of such activity is to enhance quality patient care.[38]

Some models do exist for creating a "protective zone" for reporting, discussing, and analyzing such information. Although some are found outside the health care field, most notably in the field of aviation safety, there are some models in the health care field.[39] For example, a limited peer review immunity was created by Congress in the Health Care Quality Improvement Act (HCQIA).[40] This law creates a limited immunity from damages for those who take part in peer review activities that may culminate in a health care facility's taking action against an individual's medical staff privileges. The HCQIA also affords protection to those who provide information to bodies that review data that lead to corrective action. However, even this protection has its limitations. It does not apply if the action was taken without granting the individual due process, such as a right to notice and a hearing. Moreover, if the action was not premised on the reasonable belief that it would further quality health care, such activity is not covered by the HCQIA.

The U.S. Food and Drug Administration (FDA) operates adverse event reporting systems:

> The Vaccine Adverse Event Reporting System, a program cosponsored with the Centers for Disease Control and Prevention (CDC). This

system, which started in 1990, is used to collect and analyze data from reports of adverse events following immunization. The intent is to use the system to identify new safety concerns. It is important to note that anyone can report to this system.

The Special Nutritional Adverse Event Monitoring System, a voluntary reporting system established in 1993 to address adverse events associated with use of a special nutritional product: dietary supplements, infant formulas, and medical foods.

The Manufacturer and User Facility Device Experience Database, which aggregates information on medical device adverse events.

Other federal agencies also collect information that deals with adverse events, such as the CDC's National Nosocomial Infections Surveillance System, a voluntary effort that began in 1970 between the CDC and acute care general hospitals to collect information for a national nosocomial infections database. Under applicable law, information provided by participating hospitals that would link data with any individual or institution is held in strict confidence.

At the state level, a variety of laws are designed to provide evidentiary protection for data or activities geared to peer review. The basic premise of such legislation is to create a "protective zone" in which frank and candid discourse can occur without fear that the discussions of the data reviewed will be subject to legal process. In other words, those who take part in the proceedings, whether as members of a peer review committee or as a witness, are protected from legal recourse.[41]

Many state laws were created to facilitate implementation of the HCQIA. The scope of these laws is quite narrow, applicable to hospitals and other facilities with a peer review mechanism and a due process system focused on medical staff members.[42] The laws were designed to encourage quality patient care. Written at a time when the focal point was peer review for purposes of credentialing, the laws were not designed to address root cause analysis or disclosure of unanticipated outcome information.

Although there are federal models in place for revealing adverse events without concern that such information will be used outside the scope of the reporting laws, the same cannot be said of disclosure of unanticipated outcomes of care. There are specific frameworks in place for voluntary reporting of medical device or vaccination issues. The same cannot be said for telling a patient or a family about an untoward event.

The legal concern is quite simple. If a hospital or a physician voluntarily discloses unanticipated outcome information, does this action signify a decision to give up evidentiary protection for other purposes, such as a legal proceeding for professional liability or disciplinary action before a regulatory body? Does it signify an admission of liability?

The plaintiffs' bar may well argue that by disclosing unanticipated outcome information outside the scope of peer review, the health care facility consciously relinquished evidentiary protection. The same kind of argument would be used with respect to a physician's sharing such news outside the realm of the peer review process. Although such disclosure may be required by JCAHO standards, the plaintiff may insist that such a step signifies voluntarily giving up any evidentiary protection.

The plaintiffs' bar is likely to go one step further, insisting that disclosure of unanticipated outcome or bad news is tantamount to an admission of culpability. Not only is this a specious argument, it flies in the face of the basic foundations of consent law (see Chapter Two).

The fact that a physician or a hospital spokesperson talks with the patient or family about an unanticipated outcome does not signify relinquishment of evidentiary protection. A patient and family expect to have closure in the communication process that begins with consent to treatment and ends with the outcome of a test or treatment intervention. It is curious that the plaintiffs' bar does not make such assertions when the outcome of care disclosure focuses on positive, not negative, results. Furthermore, it is expected that to complete the consent cycle, the patient and, when appropriate, the family will receive information about the tests or treatment. This is important for purposes of follow-up care, watching for side effects, or the recurrence of symptoms. Absent such information, the patient could undertake activities or consume medication that may have a negative impact on his or her health. Without such details, important warning signals about changes in health status could be ignored, to the detriment of the patient's well-being. The failure of a physician to communicate such information could be seen as substandard care. Hence, the notion that outcomes disclosure is a special communication process that relinquishes evidentiary process is unrealistic. It is incongruent with the law of consent to treatment.

To be certain, steps should be taken to make sure that well-intentioned statements about the outcomes of care are not taken out of context or that such disclosures are not seen as voluntarily relinquishment of desired evidentiary protection. Such steps include delineating a thoughtful outcomes disclosure process. Thus, patients and families can receive cogent, factual outcomes information, without blame or fault attributed to someone. It means that outcomes information can be explained so that patients and families understand that some occurrences take place without someone being at fault.

Another solution is to look for a legislative answer, ideally at the national level, to make it clear that such information, if disclosed to patients and their families, does not signal relinquishment of evidentiary protection. Legislation would encourage greater discussion without fear of recrimination for doing so. Some federal legislators are considering such an approach with a view to encouraging greater internal review of bad outcomes to enhance patient safety.[43] Until such steps are taken, it is important for health care providers to obtain practical legal advice regarding their responsibilities in the disclosure of information about unanticipated outcomes of care.

CONCLUSION

Many complex factors have helped make it difficult for caregivers to disclose information about adverse outcomes of care. Some of these complexities stem from outdated laws and outmoded legal reasoning. Against this backdrop is a groundswell of demands from consumers, payers, and accrediting bodies insisting that caregivers disclose such information. The problem is all the more difficult since most health professionals have not received training in how to interact with patients or their families in difficult circumstances.

The consent process, a topic discussed in the next chapter, provides a framework for delivering bad news or unanticipated outcomes of care. Fundamental to this process is a strong understanding of the physician-patient and physician-family relationships. The right set of skills for managing "how to say it" is essential.

CHAPTER 2

Consent as a Process

The fundamental elements for a valid informed consent process are the same whether the test or treatment involves obstetrics, oncology, or cardiology. What is different, however, are the context and the dynamics. Whereas oncology, cardiology, and other specialties are focused on the treatment or prevention of disease, obstetrics is geared to bringing a new life into the world. Pregnancy does incur risks, but the rewards go beyond those found in curing a disease or arresting cancer. Pregnancy is a time of excitement and expectation, the evolution of life plans and dreams. It marks a time of tremendous change in the life of the parents. When pregnancies culminate in happy, uncomplicated delivery outcomes, the process becomes part of a family's memory treasure chest. Quite the opposite response occurs when delivery outcomes are evidenced by tragically impaired lives or mortality of neonates.

THE CLINICAL BENEFITS OF THE CONSENT PROCESS

The consent process in obstetrics can play a pivotal role in helping set the expectations of the mother and spouse or significant other. The consent process, and in particular the history-taking phase, can be used to pinpoint risk factors previously unknown to the caregiver. Such information may lead to a change in care plans or to more time and attention being given to sharing risk information with the patient.

As a communications tool, the consent process can be used to deliver cautionary or risk information during certain periods of gestation. And it can be used as the backdrop for sharing the news about unanticipated outcomes of obstetric care. Using the consent process in this way requires a practical working knowledge not only of the basic components; it also requires a keen sense of how and when to deliver information.

Consent as a Process, Not a Form

One of the key misunderstandings of consent is that it is seen as an administrative task or another form that must be completed to satisfy the law or to obtain reimbursement for the delivery of obstetric services. Nothing can be further from reality. Consent is a process, *not* a form.[1] If anything, consent is a communications process between caregiver and patient that culminates in a decision regarding the parameters of an obstetric care plan. The consent form provides a written historical record of the agreed-on terms of care.

In some states, signed or written consent forms are viewed as providing evidence of consent.[2] In other jurisdictions, a properly completed consent form creates a "rebuttal presumption" of a valid treatment authorization.[3] In essence, the law in these states treats or presumes that the signed consent form is evidence of a successfully completed consent process. For the patient to overcome this presumption, she must present evidence to refute it. In these jurisdictions, such refuting evidence might be that the patient had received so much pain medication that when participating in the consent process, she could not have understood what she was authorizing in obstetric care. Another illustration might be that there is other written evidence that shows the requisite elements of the consent process had not been completed prior to the patient's signing the treatment authorization.

The key point is this: a form cannot replace the give and take, the dialogue, or the eye contact between health care professional and obstetric patient. Similarly, interactive consent processes found in computer software cannot serve as a substitute for important discussions about care plan options in obstetrics. If anything, such sophisticated forms are assistive tools, designed to facilitate the dialogue between caregiver and patient, not replace it.

The Foundation of the Caregiver-Patient Relationship

The consent process becomes the concrete foundation for the future direction of the caregiver-patient relationship. If a nurse midwife or an obstetrician gets off on the wrong foot with a patient or the patient's partner, it can have a chilling effect on the quality of the caregiver-patient relationship. One or the other may be reluctant to share salient information, foreclosing the possibility of effective communication for fear of jeopardizing what little rapport had been established.

It is imperative that a caregiver and an obstetric patient establish an open dialogue. It is equally important for the care provider to get to know what is important to the individual. An understanding of the dynamics of the patient's life, choices, and preferences can help shape obstetric care plans. During and after the delivery process, knowing what is important may also prove useful, especially if there is an unanticipated outcome. The consent process therefore becomes the foundation for building the rapport between caregiver and patient.

A Communication Tool Geared to Quality Patient Care

The flow of information generated by the consent process can help improve patient care and increase the chances of positive outcomes. This is particularly relevant in obstetrics in which medical history, prior challenges in pain management during labor, or previous problem pregnancy information may influence the design of the patient's care plan.

Without a good rapport, communication can prove difficult. If the caregiver does not know how to talk with a patient, the quality of the dialogue may suffer. For example, if a patient has limited English proficiency, using monosyllabic terms or speaking slowly may prove useless in effecting a successful communication. In this situation, using the resources of a qualified interpreter can enhance the quality of the dialogue, along with the opportunity for quality obstetric care.

THE CORE ELEMENTS OF CONSENT

Although the law varies from jurisdiction to jurisdiction, the basic elements of consent to treatment are essentially the same.[4] The root premise is that the patient should be provided with sufficient information to make a treatment choice. The goal of the law on the topic, whether it comes from legislation, regulation, or case law, is that the individual should be able to make an informed choice.

The law generally recognizes a set of basic elements that must be in place for a valid consent to treatment:

A discussion of the indications for tests or treatment. The patient should be apprised of the reasons for recommended tests or treatment and the bearing this has on the obstetric care plan.

A description of the nature and purpose of recommended tests or treatment. The patient should be given an understandable explanation of what is involved in a recommended diagnostic test, such as an ultrasound or alpha fetal protein testing, or obstetric treatment.

A description of the probable benefits and probable risks of recommended tests or treatment. In the therapeutic context, it is not expected that the patient should be apprised of every known risk in obstetrics or, for that matter, every known benefit. Rather, the requirement is to provide salient or significant information that would likely sway a person's decision making when selecting among a number of treatment options.

A discussion of diagnostic or treatment alternatives, if any exist, along with the attendant probable benefits and probable risks of these options. Obstetric patients are entitled to receive understandable information about alternative tests or treatment. This would include tests or treatment that may be either more aggressive or conservative than that recommended initially. The idea is to present the patient with options from which to make a treatment choice.

A description of the consequences of forgoing recommended or alternative tests or treatment. Patients need to know the likely outcomes that attend a decision to refuse a recommended or alternative diagnostic or therapeutic intervention. If, for example, an obstetric patient wants to try an alternative or complementary therapy that has no documented efficacy, the patient should be apprised of this information.

Remote risks involving paralysis, serious impairment, or death should be disclosed to the patient. When an obstetric intervention may result in a catastrophic outcome, such as paralysis, disabling stroke, or death, the patient is entitled to receive this information. However, it is incumbent on the caregiver to put the risk in a context that the patient can understand. Giving the patient statistical information is usually frowned on because it does not provide a framework within which the person can make a treatment choice. What is meant by "putting it in context"? An illustration helps to develop this point. Assume that there is a remote but nonetheless serious risk that a patient could suffer permanent nerve damage from an epidural block. To put it in a framework the patient can understand, a good approach is to say, "There is a far greater likelihood that you could win the lottery than experience nerve damage from the epidural block." Taking this step gives the patient a context in which she can appreciate what is the chance that the known, remote risk might occur.

LEGAL ABILITY AND MENTAL CAPABILITY IN CONSENT

The law assumes that an adult, and in most instances, an emancipated minor, has the legal ability and mental capability to make a treatment decision.[5] The term *legal ability* has a particular meaning. It refers to an individual's being free from a guardian of the person. An emancipated minor is one who is able to manage his or her finances and is living away from home. In the case of a pregnant twelve year old living at home with her parents, ordinarily the teenager would not be seen as having legal ability to make treatment decisions for herself. Yet some state law may consider her legally able or empowered to make treatment decisions on behalf of her child when it is born. In the case of a mentally disabled adult with a low IQ and a court-appointed guardian, it is the guardian from whom consent to treatment would be obtained. Even in these cases, however, it may be useful to talk with and obtain information from the individual to see what she wants done in terms of obstetric care. A well-intentioned custodial guardian may not truly understand the wishes and needs of such an individual.

The term *capable* refers to a state of mental function. The question the caregiver must ask is this: Does the patient have the use of her mental faculties to make a treatment choice? A woman in the throes of a terribly painful labor contraction may not have such capability in that limited time frame. Once the contraction has subsided and her senses are not affected by the painful stimulus, she could make a treatment choice.

The fact that a patient has an epidural block does not render her automatically incapable of making a treatment decision. The caregiver must decide whether the pain management has dulled or enhanced cognitive function such that the patient can make an informed choice.

Both legal ability and functional capability are determinations that must be made on a case-by-case basis. These are core prerequisites to proceeding with a successful obstetric consent process.

PUTTING THE CORE ELEMENTS OF CONSENT INTO OPERATION

From a practical standpoint, there are other factors that can help foster a successful completion of the consent process. These are steps not found in the law; these measures reflect behaviors among successful caregivers working with obstetric patients:

 • *Give the patient sufficient time to absorb information.* Patients may be overwhelmed with too much information and unable to synthesize key details effecting the validity of an obstetric treatment decision. If the information is particularly alarming or detailed, or it involves a discussion of a host of treatment choices all with a competing level of benefit and risk, it may be prudent to have the consent discussion over time rather than in one session. It may be equally useful to refer the patient to trusted Web sites for more detailed information or to provide patient-friendly literature that can be read in a more relaxed fashion at home. This assumes, of course, that time is not of the essence and that the consent process can be divided up over two or more sessions. When divided up over time, each session should begin with a recap of the earlier discussion, confirming what the person understood during the previous conversation.

• *Encourage the patient to ask questions.* A consent process is a dialogue that requires the give and take of questions, answers, and the free flow of information. Thus, throughout the course of an obstetric consent process, the patient should be encouraged to ask questions.

• *Provide understandable answers.* One of the major pitfalls found in consent practices is the use of medical terminology to obscure emotionally charged or alarming information. Hearing the medical terminology, the patient may feel awkward or embarrassed to say that she does not understand. Not wishing to appear stupid or poorly educated, the patient may just sit there and nod at the caregiver, as if to use a physical gesture to convey the sense that she understands. Assessing how much the patient understands is part of the consent process. Some caregivers might say to the obstetric patient, "Now tell me if you don't understand what I am saying." Others may put the onus on themselves by saying, "I just want to make certain that I have been very clear. Tell me what you think you heard me describe as the benefits of this particular treatment." A patient's response that is inconsistent with the information provided is an indication of the need to reformat the dialogue at a different comprehension level.

WHAT OBSTETRIC PATIENTS NEED TO OR WANT TO KNOW

Beyond the legal requirements for a valid consent and the practical considerations of obtaining a valid authorization, there are specific topics that are important in managing pregnancies to a successful outcome and should be discussed with obstetric patients:

- The likely consequences of smoking or consuming alcohol during pregnancy
- The risk factors associated with taking over-the-counter preparations, herbal substances, and natural substances during pregnancy
- The likely consequences of noncompliance with a dietary regimen in the presence of known risk factors such as diabetes mellitis or history of high blood pressure
- The benefits of exercise during pregnancy
- Weight gain that is safe during pregnancy
- Whether this obstetrician will attend the delivery
- How long it takes to get the results of genetic testing
- The safety of taking medications prescribed by other doctors, such as allergists
- The safety of taking aspirin or other analgesics for headache or pain
- The safety of using nonprescription agents for constipation, heartburn, nausea, or related gastrointestinal upset
- The indications for a cesarean section
- The benefits and risks of epidural block
- The safety of consuming caffeine during pregnancy
- The safety of sexual relations during pregnancy
- The pros and the cons of having young children attend the delivery
- The duration of the surgery and recovery time if a cesarean section is indicated
- The amount of pain that should be anticipated following an episiotomy
- The amount of pain that should be anticipated following a cesarean section.

PRACTICAL CONSIDERATIONS OF COMMUNICATION

Successful communication between caregivers and patients is based on an effective exchange of information. Talking above the head of the patient, speaking in generalities, or not disclosing significant benefit and risk information can thwart a successful consent communication.

There are other factors to consider as well. These include the use of effective interpreters and culturally sensitive communications. One common question is the propriety of having a family member or friend serve as an interpreter. Without knowing the capability of the individual to serve as the interpreter of medical information, the caregiver is relying on an unknown third party to handle an important part of the communication process. There is concern also when the interpreter is a member of the housekeeping or clinical staff who has not been tested for clinical competency to act in this capacity.

Some states have laws on the topic of interpreter services.[6] The Office of Civil Rights of the U.S. Department of Health and Human Services has issued guidance on the topic.[7] There is also case law on the requirement to accommodate patients and surrogate decision makers who require interpretive services for the hearing impaired.[8]

What the law and guidance suggest is a reasoned approach to the use of interpreters to effect solid communication. Thus, if a pregnant woman is hearing impaired and communication must be accomplished through the use of American Sign Language (ASL), the obstetric practice must accommodate the patient need. This does not mean, however, that the practice must retain the services of an ASL interpreter who charges $150 hour when a technically competent competitor is available at the rate of $50. In other words, the patient cannot insist on the high-charging interpreter when a more reasonably priced alternative can be used to accomplish effective communication.

Another practical consideration in consent communications is cultural sensitivity. Once again, the federal government has issued guidance on the subject, a reflection perhaps that the United States is continuing to be a melting pot of people from a myriad of cultures.[9] This is a topic of particular relevance in obstetric communications.

Some cultures have a strong opposition to male physicians' or nurses' providing urogenital services to women. This includes prenatal services and labor and delivery care. Having a chaperon in attendance will not overcome this cultural demand. In some instances, it may go in a different direction, in which the spouse of the pregnant woman insists on being the "spokesperson" in all consent and health care communication with the patient. In other words, the patient cannot speak for herself. This can be a serious concern, especially if the spouse as intermediary is unable to impart salient information. The same would be true if the patient holds back communicating important details out of fear of reprisal by her husband or other male intermediary.

The law requires reasonable accommodation. When an impasse occurs, it is often useful to enlist the services of a respected leader of the cultural group to facilitate an acceptable solution. Sometimes caregivers of the same culture may be able to achieve the same goal. In other instances, referral of the case to a health care facility ethics committee may be warranted. The goal is to achieve a reasonable, practical approach to a difficult communication problem.

COMMON EXCEPTIONS TO THE RULES OF CONSENT

There are a handful of well-recognized exceptions to the general rules of consent. Knowing how to manage these exceptions will help to avoid liability risk exposure based on lack of informed consent.

The common exceptions are found in statutes, regulations, and case law.[10] Although the specifics of each exception vary by state, many share a number of similarities. Therefore, it is important to become familiar with the requirements in a specific jurisdiction rather than relying on a general description of any of the exceptions.

Emergency

The law recognizes a so-called implied consent to treatment in an emergency situation.[11] An emergency in this context has a very specific connotation, referring to a situation in which a patient presents with a life- or health-threatening illness, injury, or event. The patient is unable to participate in the decision-making process. This incapacity may be due to the illness or injury, or it may be attributed to an underlying condition. The situation is so critical that there is no time to secure a treatment authorization from someone else recognized at law as having the authority to make such determinations on behalf of the patient. The law implies the consent of the patient, in essence saying that if the person were capable of making a treatment choice, he or she would readily do so.

The emergency exception applies only to tests, treatment, and surgical interventions necessary to eliminate the life- or health-threatening event. For example, an emergency may occur when a pregnant woman at full term presents with a gunshot wound to her abdomen. Unconscious, in a life-threatening state, and needing immediate surgery, the emergency team can take such steps as are necessary to save the woman's life. Doing an emergency cesarean section as part of life-saving care would come under the emergency exception. However, removal of a perfectly normal-looking appendix would constitute unauthorized treatment. Going beyond the scope of the emergency exception may trigger a claim for battery.

Impracticality of Consent

Less well recognized is a variation of the emergency exception. It addresses situations in which a patient is experiencing a life- or health-threatening event. The patient requires immediate attention, but unlike the emergency exception, is capable of taking part in the consent dialogue. However, given the urgency in such cases, there is no time to go through all the requisite elements of the consent process. Instead, key data are obtained from the patient, and treatment proceeds to eliminate the life- or health-threatening event. For example, a woman with a breech baby presents in premature labor at a hospital emergency department. She has progressed too far in labor to warrant an intervention to stop the premature delivery. The fetus also manifests signs of distress. Rather than going through the entire obstetric consent process, the caregiver uses a condensed version, explaining that the woman will soon deliver, that labor has progressed well beyond the point where attempts should be made to stop the process, and that to protect the health of the baby, it may be necessary to perform a cesarean section. In doing this urgent preparation for the premature delivery, there may be a few key questions to elicit patient history, serious risk factors, medication history, and allergy information. The questions are designed to evoke brief, and often yes or no, answers.

The "impracticality of consent" exception is applicable only to the life- or health-threatening event. It prohibits performing procedures that are not covered by the exception. Expanding treatment beyond the permissible bounds may lead to a claim of battery.

Therapeutic Privilege

Situations occur in which disclosure of consent information may cause more harm than good. A patient with an underlying psychiatric or emotional problem may be at risk to experience psychogenic shock or an exacerbation of severe depression were the individual to receive such sensitive information. The dilemma for caregivers is what to do in such cases. Should they withhold the information from the patient?

The law has fashioned a response that permits the caregiver to refrain from disclosing the threatening information. However, it does not prevent the caregiver from going through an otherwise complete consent process. To use this exception, a caregiver typically requests a consultation with a mental health specialist who is not otherwise involved in the care of the patient. The consultation may be completed by a psychiatrist or a clinical psychologist. The evaluation is focused on whether it is appropriate to invoke the therapeutic privilege exception. The results are documented in the patient record. If the consulting specialist concurs, the caregiver goes through the consent process without discussing the information that is the subject of the exception. The patient record reflects what was discussed with the patient and the details of what information was withheld during the consent process. At a later time in treatment, the information may be revealed to the patient, along with an explanation regarding why therapeutic privilege was used in the course of care.

The exception must be used very prudently. Withholding information in such cases may be seen as a way to manipulate a patient into agreeing to treatment that otherwise she or he would decline. Having the consultation from an independent specialist is seen as helping overcome such a risk factor.

Patient Refusal

Another common exception recognizes the right to refuse to be informed when making a treatment choice.[12] In essence, the patient is saying, "Look doctor, I trust you, so just go ahead and do what you think is right."

These "refusal to be informed" cases can be fraught with serious risk. It means that there is an absence of common understanding or common ground between caregiver and patient. It means that as procedures are done in the course of labor and delivery, the patient may become frightened or bewildered because of an absence of a context for why steps are being taken during treatment. Moreover, it may be a signal that the person is frightened or does not want to share information with the caregiver that would likely trigger further tests or disclosure of embarrassing information.

It is prudent to look at individuals who refuse to be informed as at-risk patients. In obstetrics, this means patients at risk for excessive expectations of care or patients at risk for complications due to a paucity of key information. The question is whether there is a way to overcome such a stalwart attitude. The answer is yes, as the following example shows:

M.H., who is seventeen weeks' pregnant, tells the nurse practitioner and the obstetrician that she agrees to all routine care and adds, "Just give me the papers to sign." When the nurse practitioner and the obstetrician attempt to discuss with her the pros and cons of a care plan, she interrupts and says, "Look, I told you: just give me the papers to sign. I don't have time for all this medical gibberish. Just do what you have to do, okay?" Despite another attempt to discuss the care plan, she says, "I am telling you I don't want to hear all about it. Just let me sign the darn papers!"

Rather than accommodate her, the obstetrician changes tactics and says, "M.H., I understand what you are saying. You can request to have treatment without our discussing with you the pros and cons of certain measures in the pregnancy care plan. But I am uncomfortable doing so, and here is where I am coming from. You are as much a part of the health care team as I am. We need a strong working relationship, and that includes an open line of communication. I need to know what makes you tick. I need to know your preferences, your medical history, and things of that nature. Without having that information, it is like my trying to drive a car in a really dense fog. It is simply not safe. And I won't drive that car in a dense fog. So what I am saying to you is this: you can have your treatment without being informed, but I won't be part of the caregiving team. I will work with you to find an obstetrician who is comfortable with this situation. But I would rather work with you by discussing the pros and cons in a way that doesn't unduly alarm you or get you to discuss things that are uncomfortable for you. So why don't you take a few minutes to think this idea over, and I will come back and visit with you."

After M.H. has had some time to absorb what the doctor has suggested, she agrees to participate in the consent process. They hammer out a rapport and an approach to communication that is comfortable for both of them. In addition, the doctor documents in the patient record what he told M.H.

The lesson learned here is this: sometimes a "frontal attack" with what caregivers believe is routine information creates a communication obstacle. When a patient says no to receiving information, that is the patient's prerogative. However, an important threshold consideration is finding out why the patient is reluctant to participate in the discussion, address that issue first, and then move on to the consent process.

PRACTICAL ISSUES IN OBSTETRICS CONSENT

A host of practical concerns come up in the course of the obstetric consent process. Knowing that these issues are likely to be on the table for discussion, caregivers can anticipate patient concerns and furnish such information without first being asked to do so. This demonstrates to the patient that the caregiver has given a lot of thought to what is important to her.

In terms of supplying such information, it may be done through a dialogue or perhaps a brochure entitled, *Frequently Asked Questions in Obstetric Care: What Patients Want to Know*. The fact that the document was given to the patient should be recorded in the patient record. Many health care facilities and medical practices use this approach. Many end their brochure with a paragraph that encourages the patient to ask questions. This is important too, since a brochure may not resolve concerns or issues that the individual may have about her care plan. That these questions were asked and that the caregiver responded to these outstanding issues should be noted in the patient record.

Whether addressed in a brochure, a videotape, or an informational Web site, there are common questions, responses, and standard information that patients should receive in the course of the obstetric consent process.

Is It Just the Patient or Patient and Partner Who Should Be Part of the Process?

The law looks to the caregiver-patient relationship as the foundation for the consent process. It sets a baseline standard for all patients. As such, it does not share the practical vision of health care entities and professionals who readily understand that the contemporary consent process is one in which it is better to engage family members or partners in the dialogue rather than relegating them to a waiting room. The practical reality is that having a baby is a shared experience involving the patient, father, and extended family. With the permission of the patient, having the others involved serves several purposes. First, it opens the line of communication with family members who may be able to shed light on family history unknown to the patient, information that can be important to the care plan. Second, it creates a team effort for helping the patient get through her pregnancy. With a noncompliant patient, having a group of coaches helping her stay the course is far better than dealing with the aftermath of care plan noncompliance. Third, it creates a relationship with people who may be the recipients of adverse outcome information. Knowing them beforehand means that there is a relationship or existing personal dynamic in which to discuss bad news. Hence, for all these reasons, it is better to involve others in the consent process from the outset. The key is to secure the patient's authorization to do so. Once a member of the care team, the family member or partner must be made to understand his or her role and responsibility, including keeping health care information confidential.

Is Obstetrics a Partnership Between Caregiver and Patient?

One aspect of patient care shared by chronically ill individuals and pregnant women is the importance of forging a strong working relationship with their caregivers. Many patients see their caregiver only for routine annual visits or when they have a serious ailment; these infrequent interactions create a different rapport from that found between patients and obstetric caregivers who work with one another on a regular basis.

The obstetric experience benefits when the caregiver and the patient understand each other's roles and responsibilities. The successful relationship is founded on trust and solid communication. The communication begins with the consent process in which the caregiver maps out his or her expectation of the relationship, including the importance of sharing information and how to contact the caregiver.

The relationship can be strained when something untoward occurs, such as a miscarriage or unanticipated complication. However, it may not be wrenched apart if the relationship is premised on trust and communication. Hence, a key part of the introduction to the obstetric care plan is to discuss what the patient should do and, in appropriate cases, what the family or partner can do to facilitate a working relationship.

Why Is Patient History So Important?

Patient history information, or the absence of it, can play a pivotal role in the successful management of a pregnancy. Knowing about key risk factors in terms of personal or family history may trigger the need for consults with specialists in endocrinology, immunology, urology, or cardiology. Having risk information in hand from the outset means that the care plan is geared to a patient-specific outcome. An obstetrician or perinatologist potentially can use the history information to avert serious risks or minimize the opportunity for problems to occur during the pregnancy. In essence, medical history taking becomes a core ingredient in obstetric patient safety.

During the consent process, the caregiver has a unique opportunity to obtain important patient history. Doing so, however, requires more than asking broadly worded questions. Incumbent on the caregiver is the need to ask "drill down" questions that get to the core of medical history that can shed light on serious obstetric risk factors. To achieve this purpose, the caregiver should explain to the patient why it is so important to be honest and to respond to all questions, even those that may seem unrelated or embarrassing. A skilled clinician asks follow-up questions to make certain that the information is accurate and consistent with details learned in the course of obtaining the patient history.

What Is Meant by Material or Significant Information?

In the therapeutic context, the law does not require caregivers to provide information on all known benefits or risks associated with recommended treatment. Rather, the law requires that the caregiver provide "material" or "significant" information.[13] Jurisdictions differ on whether materiality or significance of information should be measured by the standard of the medical community or the reasonable patient.[14] Notwithstanding this difference of opinion, there remains the basic question of what is material or significant information.

The law has provided little guidance on the subject. Instead, it may defer to an expert opinion, guidelines from a recognized medical group, or a standard of practice. From the patient perspective, what patients consider material or significant may not be consistent with the perception of caregivers on the topic.

Leaving aside the legal requirements, there are practical considerations that help to give shape to the scope of the information that should be imparted in the consent process. Some take a broad approach asking, "If you were in the patient's position, what would you like to be told to make your choice an informed decision?" In other instances, it is more specific, including an articulation about such risks as alcohol, tobacco, and medication use during pregnancy; the pros and cons of various forms of pain management; the use of cesarean section versus vaginal birth; the risks of sexual relations during pregnancy; and the chief problems that might occur during pregnancy, such as diabetes mellitus, hypertension, or related issues.

Caregivers need to set a norm for their practices. Dialogues with patients about material or significant information should take into consideration religious, cultural, and ethnocentric practices of patients. Listening to and learning from patients, care providers can identify the type of information that is considered particularly important or useful in formulating a treatment decision. Following the lead of their patients, what is recommended by national professional organizations, and the requirements of applicable law, caregivers can develop a practical framework for what is considered material or significant information.

Does the Consent Process Occur in Stages?

The communication dialogue between caregiver and patient is often a process that occurs over time and at various stages of the treatment process. This is particularly true for those who require care for cancer, chronic ailments, dialysis, or pregnancy. As the underlying conditions change, and the risks and benefits change, or new modalities are needed, so too is there a need for a refreshing of the consent process to accommodate the circumstances.

In other instances, the information may be so complex or alarming that from a strategic perspective, it is better to divide it up into consent sessions rather than trying to deliver the details in one encounter. For example, if an obstetric patient is carrying a fetus that has a potentially life-threatening defect and the mother is always apprehensive, it may be prudent to use the consent session approach: rather than overwhelming the patient with detailed information in one session, spacing it out may make it easier for her to synthesize the information in order to make a treatment choice. The sessions may occur over the course of several hours or a few days. When this approach is used, it is important to document in the patient record when each session occurred and who was present and to summarize the information provided to the patient.

Is It Useful to Check Along the Way to Confirm Patient Understanding Throughout the Pregnancy?

One step that is often missing in the consent process is an affirmation that the caregiver and the patient have the same understanding of what is involved in the care plan, a specific procedure, or a treatment alternative. The same is true for patient self-care requirements, including the medication regimen, when to contact the clinician, or when to seek urgent medical assistance during the pregnancy.

It is not enough to include in the consent form a statement to the effect that "Ms. J. understood the nature and purpose of the planned cesarean section based on her answers to questions posed about the procedure." The affirmation question-and-answer session must take place.

The process can be done very easily. For example, the physician might say, "Okay, Ms. J., I wanted to be certain that we are both on the same page in terms of what we are going to be doing next Thursday. Tell me what you understand about the procedure." If Ms. J.'s response is inconsistent with what was articulated during the consent process, it is a risk management indicator that there is a communications problem. It is time to retool the explanation until the patient is able to respond with an appropriate answer.

Should a Physician Rely on Common Knowledge as Part of the Obstetric Consent Process?

Common knowledge refers to health care information that a health care professional can assume is within the frame of reference of the average patient. Examples include taking aspirin to reduce a temperature or seeking medical attention if someone has severe chest pain. In essence, the law assumes that the average reasonable person "knows" such information and that such knowledge may have been acquired through reading newspapers or news magazines, watching television, listening to radio programs, or surfing health care Web sites.

The practical issue is that two average patients may not have the same framework for general health care information. Much depends on the person's experience and exposure to sources that provide this information. Thus, relying on what one assumes a patient knows is like trying to steer a ship through a dense fog. There is no frame of reference or starting point. A seasoned ship's captain may be able to make a good estimate of his vessel's position and avoid running aground. Similarly, the seasoned obstetrician may make a good assumption about how much she can depend on the degree of common knowledge the patient has about obstetrics. But if the assumption is wrong and the patient does not receive the benefit of information disclosure, the result could be an inadequate consent process.

Relying on the idea of common knowledge is like a game of Russian roulette. Some will win; others will not. Such risk-taking behavior is incongruent with quality patient care. The better approach is not to rely on assumptions and to validate patient understanding by means of a series of questions that are designed to test knowledge of material or significant information needed for quality obstetric care.

Reliance on common knowledge is fraught with risk. It can be an expedient used to rush the consent process. It can overlook the challenges of patients with communication deficits, including those for whom English is a second language. It overlooks the fact that depending on where one grew up or resides now, idioms and local parlance regarding common health information may have a meaning entirely different from that ascribed to the constellation of mainstream common knowledge in obstetrics. Hence, taking into consideration all of these issues, the more prudent approach is not to rely on common knowledge in the obstetric consent process.

Can a Caregiver Use the Consent Process to Modulate Expectations?

Patients and their partners can develop excessive expectations easily in terms of the outcome of the pregnancy. Some caregivers describe it as a phenomenon in which the patient hears what she wants to hear. Others see it as patients getting caught up in the groundswell of wanting and expecting a healthy baby.

The consent process can be a useful tool in adjusting expectations of care. The back-and-forth dialogue gives the caregiver an opportunity to evaluate patient desires, needs, and expectations. Patients with excessive expectations are at risk for communication problems based on unrealistic beliefs about treatment outcome. Anything less than what they expect may result in acrimony or, worse, litigation.

On a radio, the volume control is used to adjust how loud music is played. The consent process can function in a similar fashion. The dialogue of the consent process can be used to adjust inordinate expectations of care.

What Do I Say?

When such an issue is identified, this fact is documented in the patient record along with a summary of what the caregiver said to put outcome expectations in perspective with the patient and, when applicable, with her partner.

Can a Patient Revoke Her Consent During the Labor and Delivery Process?

Caregivers often ask whether they have to respect the wishes of a patient who changes her mind during labor and delivery and revokes her consent to a particular treatment modality. The answer depends on a number of factors.

The general rule is that caregivers should respect the right of the patient to say no to treatment or to withdraw an authorization of previously agreed-on care. The assumption is that when the patient decides she does not want a cesarean section, she has the requisite mental ability to make such a decision. If, for example, the pain management administered to the woman leaves her incoherent and unable to identify date and place, it may be prudent to do a consent capability evaluation. This may be done by a specialist in behavioral health care, such as a clinical psychologist or psychiatrist. If time is of the essence, it may be necessary for the obstetrician to make a professional judgment call, perhaps in concert with the attending anesthesiologist. They may assess the patient's cognitive faculties and decide that given her inability to respond correctly to simple questions, recognizing the amount of pain medication she has received and the recognized effect it has on patients, she lacks the requisite ability at the time to make a treatment decision. This extends to revocation of consent to previously agreed-on obstetric care.

If the patient has the requisite ability to revoke her consent, the decision should be an informed choice. In many instances, however, obstetricians and perinatologists do not have the luxury of time to go through the nuances of such a choice. Instead, they are faced with time-sensitive decision making that requires disclosure of material benefit and risk information and the consequences of revoking consent to previously planned care. When a decision finally is made, the patient record should reflect the fact that the patient was informed of the consequences of revoking her consent and that in doing so, it had been determined that she had the requisite cognitive ability to do so.

If the revocation of consent takes place earlier in the pregnancy and the caregiver is uncomfortable carrying on with treatment of the patient, a decision has to be made how to handle the case. The caregiver cannot simply walk away from the individual once the treatment relationship has begun. Instead, the caregiver should talk to the patient and explain why he or she cannot continue to provide obstetric services. The caregiver should offer to help the individual find another health care professional willing to treat the patient on her terms. The discussion should be handled carefully so that it does not appear that the caregiver is trying to force the patient to change her mind through intimidation or coercion. Regardless of the state in which a doctor or nurse practices, the law takes a dim view of coercion or duress. Such tactics actually can nullify an otherwise valid consent process. The patient record should reflect the fact that the discussion took place, and a summary should be included of the efforts taken to find another caregiver. This is an important step in the event that the patient later files a complaint for abandonment.

Another common problem involves a change of mind after the point of no return has been reached in the caregiving process. For example, if a patient agreed to a cesarean section and two-thirds of the way into the procedure she "changes her mind," it is in practical terms too late for a revocation of consent. The patient record should nevertheless reflect the fact that this turn of events took place and how the caregiver handled it in terms of communicating with the patient.

Revocation of consent is a signal that there may be a problem in the communication process. It means that with further dialogue with the patient, the reason may surface for the revocation of consent, and it can be addressed without the patient's declining necessary care or embarking on a precarious course of treatment.

Should a Caregiver Use Duress or Coercion to Address Problems in Obstetric Consents?

The quiver of acceptable communication skills should not include duress or coercion. Patients should never be presented with a take-it-or-leave-it approach to the delivery of obstetric services. When patients request services that cannot be accommodated, they should be apprised of this fact. However, they should not be subjected to coercion, threats, or intimidation that make them accede to a standardized protocol that is contrary to their cultural or religious beliefs. Similarly, threatening to call in social services, a state agency, or the police are tactics that should never be used to secure consent to treatment. Such an approach is coercive and outside the established norm for consent communication.

The use of duress or coercion can vitiate or nullify the consent process. The use of such tactics can lead to complaints, litigation, and, in some instances, allegations of unprofessional conduct in which the caregiver's license or registration may be at risk. The onus of adverse publicity in such cases can be hard to overcome as well. Thus, the prudent approach is to avoid using such methods to make the patient reach a treatment decision.

CONSENT AS A PATIENT SAFETY TOOL IN OBSTETRICS

Obstetric consent procedures play a pivotal role in terms of risk management and patient safety. The "drill-down" approach to asking clear, understandable questions, confirmatory questions, and testing patient understanding of agreed-on treatment are all steps that help identify potential clinical risk factors. Once these risk factors are known, caregivers can design treatment plans that help avoid such risk exposures.

As a patient safety tool, the obstetric consent process helps to identify the patient's responsibility for avoiding known risk factors. For example, if a pregnant woman has an underlying kidney ailment, alerting her to the signs of potential risk factors enables her to take swift action should such a problem emerge. If the patient has granted permission for a family member or partner to participate in the consent process, the family can be equipped with the informational tools needed to seek help when a risk factor does appear. Knowing what to expect and what to watch for gives the patient, her partner, and family members a definite role and responsibility in the caregiver process. Reinforcing this responsibility in the course of routine or high-risk obstetric care transforms the consumer of health care services into a member of the caregiving team. It also makes the person a patient safety officer for that pregnancy.

DOCUMENTATION OF CONSENT

Although consent is a communications process, it also needs to be recorded to reflect the fact that it occurred. This is important for treatment, billing, and legal defense.

Traditionally, consent forms have been found in standardized formats. One, the so-called long form consent, details all the benefits, risks, and alternatives of a proposed obstetric test or treatment. It also captures information on the consequences of refusing care. The other type of document, the short form consent, typically has the following wording: "I [name of patient or decision maker] have received an explanation of the probable benefits, risks, and alternatives to the treatment I have authorized. I am satisfied with the explanation I have received and agree to the following [test or treatment]. [Patient's signature and date.]"

Each type of documentation has its adherents. Critics of the long form consent argue that if one fails to mention in the document a probable risk or benefit or treatment alternative, it can be used as evidence that the caregiver did not disclose such information. Others claim that the short form consent is a flawed approach since the absence of detail means that the doctor or nurse midwife must recall from memory what was discussed with the patient. Since lawsuits take time to come to court and memories fad, the danger is that the recall of the caregiver may not be sufficient to substantiate what did take place years earlier.[15]

Others frown on the use of standardized consent forms. They believe a better approach is to document the consent process by means of a detailed note in the medical record noting the key points of the consent process, including an explanation for recommended tests or treatment, a summary of the probable risks, benefits, and alternatives discussed with the patient, and the consequences of declining care. A statement is included about the patient's (or surrogate decision maker's) ability to make a treatment choice and the individual's apparent ability to understand the information. A sentence is typically included that details who was present during the consent process. The notation is then signed and dated by the caregiver.

In some institutions, a combination approach is in use, incorporating a procedure-specific consent form with the detailed note in the medical record. In addition, some obstetric practices use their own consent procedures, such as the detailed note in the office-based record, along with an accommodation for a hospital-based consent form. Many obstetric practices go further, using a paper trail approach to consent. In this case, the record would include a summary checklist of tools provided to the patient. It would also include copies of information sheets, brochures, or pamphlets provided to the patient; an indication that the patient was given an informational CD-ROM, DVD, or videotape to view; and any Web site lists provided to the patient. Any e-mail traffic on consent between the caregiver and patient would be incorporated as evidence of information used to facilitate consent. The rationale is to create a layered approach to consent, demonstrating the degree to which information was given to the patient, along with evidence of the format for disseminating it to the individual.

The detailed note approach can be time-consuming. It has the risk that the caregiver may leave out a key point of the process, triggering questions about the completeness of the consent. However, it is also the most customized consent document and thus it can have more credibility than a standard consent form.

Whether one uses a consent form, a detailed note in the record, or a checklist that delineates the informational tools provided to patients, it does remove the need for two-way communication with patients. Dialogue is critical to a successful communication process.

INNOVATION IN CONSENT DOCUMENTATION: THE CONSENT FORM FOR CAREGIVERS

An innovative approach is to develop consent tools that are for use by caregivers, not patients. The idea is to provide obstetricians, obstetric nurse practitioners, and nurse midwives with a document that prompts them to do the following:

- Establish patient ability to participate in the consent process.

- Address the need for accommodation.

- Involve family or a significant other in the consent process.

- Ask the right questions.

- Obtain an appropriate patient history.

- Share material information.

- Answer patient questions.

- Validate patient understanding of information provided during the consent process.

Special consent considerations may be part of the consent checklist—for example:

- The Emergency Medical Treatment and Active Labor Act Consent

- Allergy

- Mentally incapacitated

- Advance directives

- Limitations on care (for example, no blood or blood by-products)

- Special religious considerations

- Special cultural considerations

- Use of interpreters

At the end of the process, the consent checklist may be signed and dated by the caregiver. In this way, it becomes another layer of evidence of consent. More important, giving the caregiver a checklist from which to work lessens the need to rely on memory. It is a tool that helps facilitate completion of all the requisite steps of the obstetric consent process, and it goes further, aiding the caregiver to identify and address at-risk situations before such concerns turn into a risk management, patient safety, or liability issue.

LIABILITY EXPOSURE AND LACK OF INFORMED CONSENT TO OBSTETRIC CARE

The failure to secure obstetric consent or to do so in a substandard fashion can have legal repercussions. These include a denial of claims for reimbursement, state and federal investigation of complaints involving quality-of-care issues, and state licensing body disciplinary proceedings involving allegations of unprofessional conduct.

More common are civil lawsuits brought by aggrieved patients. In years past, consent litigation was based on intentional torts or civil wrongs in which there was no need to prove injury. Such claims are based on battery or unconsented to touching. For example, if an obstetrician administered a blood transfusion to a Jehovah's Witness patient who specifically refused such treatment for postpartum hemorrhage, this would be a battery. Although this care might save the patient's life, it still constitutes a battery. Damages can be quite high in these cases.

Lawsuits can proceed on the basis of misrepresentation, deceit, or fraud. If a caregiver consciously (intentionally) misstates risks or withholds material information in order to secure a consent that would otherwise be refused, a lawsuit may follow. Depending on the way the claim is crafted by legal counsel, the complaint may include allegations of misrepresentation, deceit, and fraud. Plaintiffs who are successful in pursuing such a claim may also be successful in obtaining punitive damages in such cases.

The most common basis for consent litigation is negligence, an unintentional tort in which actual harm must be demonstrated by the plaintiff. To be successful, the plaintiff must demonstrate:

- The standard of care related to what should have been disclosed.

- What was disclosed did not measure up to the standard of care.

- Harm to the patient was reasonably foreseeable as a consequence of the failure to abide by the standard of care.

- The patient suffered harm that was causally linked to the failure to abide by the standard of care.

In negligent consent cases, many plaintiffs fail to prove all the requisite elements of the claim. Many are able to prove a failure to provide salient information successfully. However, the requisite standard of disclosure may thwart the lawsuit. In some jurisdictions, the standard of disclosure is based on what a reasonable person in the patient's position would want to know in order to make a treatment choice. Thus, although the obstetrician failed to meet the standard of care, if the reasonable person would still have agreed to the procedure, a key component of the negligence claim is missing, and the plaintiff cannot prevail. In other jurisdictions, the standard of disclosure is based on what the medical community believes the patient needs to know. If the doctor's disclosure of information was consistent with the standard of care in the community in terms of what the physician believed the patient should know, the plaintiff would be unable to prevail in a claim based on negligent consent. This medical community standard is now a minority position. Expert witnesses usually are used to establish the standard of disclosure under either the "reasonable patient" or "medical community" standard. It should be noted that the need for expert witnesses is often a function of applicable state law.[16]

Even if the plaintiff does not prevail, a consent lawsuit can prove to be a gut-wrenching proposition for members of the health care team. It is a time-consuming, expensive process. That someone would go to the extent of filing a claim or a complaint is an indicator of a breakdown in communications. This is a risk that no one involved in obstetric care should want to accept when tools are at their disposal that can help avert litigation or administrative complaints.

THE CONSENT PROCESS AS THE INTRAVENOUS LINE OF COMMUNICATION

The consent process can be likened to an intravenous (IV) line. It is a vital part of the health care delivery process, whether the person receiving the "IV" therapy is a cancer patient or a woman about to deliver a baby. Like an intravenous line, it should not and cannot be taken for granted.

When a nurse or a physician sets up an IV line, the procedure requires meticulous attention to detail. Protocols must be followed to make certain that the line is set up successfully. Once established, the line is monitored. Sometimes the line is irrigated with fluids to keep it operating smoothly. At the first signs of trouble, interventions are made to maintain the line, and if this is not possible, a new line is established. When problems do occur, such as intravenous fluids seeping into surrounding tissue, swift action is taken to stop the seepage from causing harm.

The consent process is similar in many ways. It too requires meticulous attention to detail. Steps must be followed to make certain that the consent will be recognized as acceptable in law. As the patient's condition changes and there are shifts in benefits, risks, or the need for new treatment, there may be need for a new consent process. In those cases in which the patient is receiving repetitive health care services, such as dialysis or routine prenatal care, a "systems check" is completed to make certain that the underlying condition has not changed and warrants a new form of care or a modification to the treatment plan. Throughout the consent process, the doctor, the nurse, *and* the patient must keep patent the intravenous line of communication.

When something untoward does occur, having the preexisting IV of consent communication in place helps to facilitate the discussion of unanticipated outcomes of care. Trying to establish such a rapport in the midst of a crisis can prove difficult. Indeed, attempting to do so at that time may be as arduous as trying to set up an IV for a patient in severe shock. It is a far better approach to set up the IV as a preventive measure, ensuring a mechanism for effective communications among caregivers, patients, and their family members.

THE USE OF THE CONSENT PROCESS IN OBSTETRICS: CASE EXAMPLES

Applying the principles of consent communication makes the concepts more meaningful and useful. Through a series of examples, key components of the consent process are demonstrated that help to reinforce the ways in which communication can help avert problems in the first instance and then later serve as a context for what to say about an adverse outcome.

Managing Lifestyle Issues in Obstetric Consent

In high-risk pregnancy cases, the discussion of potential risk factors may require greater discussion. Thus, a woman with a history of multiple miscarriages merits a frank dialogue of the chance that a similar outcome may occur in this pregnancy. A patient at risk of premature birth deserves a candid discussion about the specifics of a bed rest care plan so that there is nothing left to chance or misunderstanding about the activities of daily living in which she can participate until after labor and delivery.

Lifestyle issues are important in high-risk pregnancy. Both the patient and spouse or partner need counseling on what is an acceptable activity level. Bed rest for three months can have a tremendous financial and emotional burden on all concerned. If the couple has two small children at home and the woman's salary represents a major portion of the family income, the added burden of child care expense could have severe financial consequences. Staying at rest for lengthy periods of time can lead to psychological problems and cause friction between the spouse and with other members of the family. Sexual abstinence, a medical recommendation in some cases, may add to the emotional strain of the situation.

Many caregivers do not view the consent process as providing a context for addressing these nonlegal issues. From a practical perspective, however, the consent process is a strong framework for addressing such matters. All of these issues—alcohol, drugs, bed rest, dietary modification, sex—are lifestyle issues. The ability to achieve compliance turns on several factors. Willpower is but one factor. Having accurate information, knowing about alternatives, and having ongoing support all contribute to a compliance-based treatment approach. By the same token, knowing the issues and concerns facing the patient and her family helps the caregiver develop a practical care plan. It also enables the caregiver to draw in ancillary services to assist the patient and her family during the high-risk pregnancy. Consent, the communication process, enables both sides of the equation to exchange important information that can facilitate a positive outcome. A case example illustrates this point.

J.S. and R.S. are expecting their third child. They have a boy four years of age and a girl age three. J.S. and R.S. are both gainfully employed. R.S. is a supervisor at a local precision steel grinding plant, and J.S. is an executive assistant with a local accounting firm. The family relocated to the area six months ago. They have no immediate family members within a hundred-mile radius of their home. Their respective parents are elderly and cannot provide child care assistance.

During the second trimester of pregnancy, J.S. develops serious complications. The obstetrician tells her that in order to save the pregnancy, she will need total bed rest. When he shares this news with the couple, the doctor sees that they become emotionally tense. J.S. begins to cry. Not wanting to pry, the doctor asks, "Is it simply a matter of being confined to bed, J.S., or is there more going on here? Will this treatment plan be hard to do? You know, if you talk with me, I might be able to get the right people mobilized to help you." J.S. tells the doctor that the couple's health plan will provide for a home health worker two hours per day. J.S. has no short-term disability plan, so her only recourse is to take a leave of absence from her job. The loss of her paycheck will result in a 50 percent reduction in their income. Although they have some savings, it is not enough to help them obtain needed child care for the remainder of her pregnancy. Moreover, the doctor has told the couple to expect a fairly long recovery until J.S. is able to get back up on her feet after three months of complete bed rest.

Having discussed the situation with them, the doctor realizes that the couple is facing tremendous emotional, financial, and logistical issues. He obtains their permission to enlist the aid of a medical social worker. Community-based resources are identified by the medical social worker to help get the family through the high-risk period. The result is a high compliance with the bed rest regimen and a successful pregnancy.

The case example illustrates that the consent process goes well beyond the core elements of disclosing information about potential benefits and potential risks. It encompasses a discussion of related factors that can improve or deter compliance with established treatment protocols.

Why Consent Is More Than a Piece of Paper

The consent process is not about paper forms. It is a communications tool that enables the caregiver and the patient to share key information necessary to shape a practical, appropriate care plan. The consent process enables the patient to set out her wishes, desires, needs, and concerns. Knowing this information, the caregiver can offer appropriate treatment. As a communications process, the consent discussion can help modulate excessive or unreasonable expectations of care.

A standard consent form cannot replace the richness of the dialogue between caregiver and patient or supplant the follow-up questions that flow from answers to questions posed by the caregiver. Similarly, a consent form cannot read the visual and auditory cues that the patient provides in response to questions posed by or information provided by the caregiver.

Some might ask whether there is any role for a consent form in the process. As discussed earlier in this chapter, some states require consent forms to be signed by patients. Others require written evidence of consent. Accreditation standards, such as those published by the Joint Commission on Accreditation of Healthcare Organizations, in many instances also encourage the use of signed consent documents.

A piece of paper is not a surrogate for forging a relationship between caregiver and patient, however. Nor is it a replacement for the communication that is so critical to patient care, especially in such an emotionally charged area of treatment as pregnancy.

Nevertheless, there is a role for documentation in the consent process. Well-written brochures, instruction sheets, and checklists can augment the communication process. For example, prenatal visits may include the use of update checklists, with questions designed to ask the patient how she is doing and to elicit answers that suggest when further discussion is warranted with the patient. A case example highlights this approach:

M.G. experienced three miscarriages prior to her current pregnancy. She denied consumption of alcohol or smoking during her previous pregnancies, but her obstetrician and the obstetric nurse practitioner believe that she is drinking alcohol. During her fourth-month visit, M.G. is asked to complete the update questionnaire. It begins with the following introduction: "Please take a few moments to complete this questionnaire. For us to provide you with a patient-appropriate care plan, we depend on you to provide us with honest, accurate answers." Question 12 states, "Since your last visit, how many times have you consumed alcohol or beer? 0–1, 2–4, 5–7, 8+." M.G. answers "0–1." Question 14 asks, "Have you experienced any of the following: (a) headache (b) lightheadedness (c) dizziness (d) feeling of faintness?" M.G. answers yes to 14(b) and 14(c). When called to the examining room, she asks her spouse to give the questionnaire to the nurse practitioner. When her husband scans the questionnaire, he says, "Come on, M. You know you have been drinking wine five or six times a week. Why not tell the truth? How do you expect these folks to help you?"

The questionnaire, a tool in the consent process, does not replace the dialogue between caregiver or patient. In the example provided, it triggered some issues about lightheadedness and dizziness that did not stack up with other answers that the patient provided. The intercession of the patient's spouse did help to elucidate the underlying problem to some extent. What it did not do, however, was to help the caregivers understand why M.G. decided not to be honest with them about her drinking. The revelation points to the need for additional tools to be used to help her overcome her drinking behavior during pregnancy. It also indicates that more dialogue is needed with M.G. to be certain that she understands the nature and consequences of her behavior during pregnancy.

The consent form will never replace the give-and-take exchange that is the hallmark of the caregiver-patient relationship. Documentation can be used to facilitate the process, as a tool for education, for reminding patients about appropriate behaviors, or as prompts that remind the patient when it is imperative to seek help. In the end, consent is a communications process, not a piece of paper.

The Impatient Patient

The consent process is a practical communications tool that can help galvanize the relationship between patient and caregiver. It also can serve as a vehicle for dialogue on sensitive topics with obstetric patients. The fact that the caregiver documents the process and the tools used to foster communication is important should there be a bad outcome in the case. However, the primary focus should be on using the process to help establish the relationship and use it to exchange key information with the patient. A case example illustrates this point:

> Dr. C. was running about ninety minutes behind schedule. His day had been going smoothly until 1:00 P.M., when one of his high-risk patients encountered a significant complication. Although the outcome was successful, it completely disrupted his schedule for the balance of the day. One of the patients inconvenienced by the delay was S.W.
>
> A rising star at a local Internet service provider, Ms. W. was also fanatic about timeliness. After forty-five minutes of waiting, she went to the reception desk and said, "What is going on here? Doesn't my schedule mean anything to Dr. C.? Where does he get off taking advantage of his patients like this, keeping us all waiting? Who does he think he is anyway?" She stormed out of the office and called her health plan to complain. She was not the first one from whom the health plan had received such a complaint about Dr. C.
>
> A formal quality review was launched based on six similar complaints collected over a three-month period. It turned out that there were some contributing factors to the problem. Dr. C.'s patient census had increased by 40 percent since the retirement of his partner, and he had been unsuccessful in recruiting a new associate to the practice. The office administrator had been swamped with notification to the patients of the retiring partner, and she had not focused on the escalating level of time management complaints from patients.
>
> A quality representative from the health plan reviewed the situation and suggested that the doctor *and* his office staff improve their communication strategies. She suggested the following steps:

What Do I Say?

- Provide patients with notice about the potential for unforeseeable delays due to obstetric emergencies.
- Encourage patients to call ahead to ascertain when they should arrive for their appointments.
- Be flexible and enable patients to reschedule without conflict if the office is backed up due to emergency cases.
- Monitor patient scheduling to avoid the potential for time bottlenecks.
- Handle unanticipated delays in a professional, understanding manner.
- Use hospitality-style verbal messages ("sincere apologies," for example) to defuse an irate patient, including asking the patient to meet with the office administrator or a member of the professional staff in a room away from the waiting room.
- Schedule time-sensitive patients with care, taking into consideration work hours for such patients.

In the case of Ms. W., the health plan consultant had specific advice for the doctor. She suggested that he call her and set up a time to meet with her that was consistent with Ms. W's schedule. She went further, encouraging the doctor to apologize for the delay and explain it to his patient. In doing so, she suggested that Dr. C. thank her for her help in making him realize what his scheduling problems were doing to his patients and his practice. In working with Ms. W., Dr. C. was encouraged to seek her advice on how he might accommodate her scheduling needs and to use this information in his future discussions with her about care planning and expectations. As the health plan consultant said, "Dr. C., this will be her first baby. She does not have a clue how a baby can disrupt the lifestyle of a high-powered professional. She needs a reality check that it all does not come to a grinding stop with the delivery process. It is just the beginning. And given her display in your office, use this information to do a systems check with her to make certain she has a realistic expectation of care."

The consent process is a way of identifying care management issues early in the prenatal experience. It helps to pinpoint patients who have inordinate expectations of care or difficulty in appreciating the dynamics of a baby's entering the life of the family. By using the consent process to identify and manage the expectations of the impatient patient, the caregiver can take steps to forestall complaints and, possibly, litigation.

CONCLUSION

The consent process is a systematic approach to developing and maintaining the caregiver-patient relationship in obstetrics and other medical specialties. Consent is more than the accumulation of years of case law, statutes, and regulations. It is a practical tool that helps set up a vital communications line between caregivers and patients. And it becomes the context for discussing negative outcomes with patients, their partners, and family members.

CHAPTER 3

The Challenge of Full Disclosure

The counseling strategies discussed in this book embrace a single philosophy: full disclosure of the adverse outcome and medical practices leading to that outcome should be immediate, honest, and complete and should not be influenced by the nature of the adverse outcome.

THE VALUE OF FULL DISCLOSURE

Young care providers may reject the concept of full disclosure on many levels. Admitting error might be perceived as a sign of weakness or inadequacy. Such admissions of responsibility, they believe, surely will lead to increases in lawsuits. Doesn't it take more energy to be so forthright? (Here, the seasoned care provider would say it takes more energy to conceal issues than it does to be forthcoming with all of the facts.) And won't such admissions make the care provider feel inadequate, a failure, and fearful? They even may ask, "Why would anyone want to weaken the physician-patient relationship by such honest statements?"

More seasoned care providers recognize the value of full disclosure, even in today's litigious medical environment. This form of acknowledgment begins by understanding our role as care providers. As a simple metaphor, the medical course that the patient experiences is likened to travel on a train. Our role as care providers is more that of a conductor rather than the object of the journey. We assist in the process and therefore must not mistake our role instead to be the object of the process. By defining ourselves as process oriented instead of only goal oriented, we replace "win at all costs" with "I am here to assist." As such, we recognize the centrist role played by our patient and her medical course.

For each patient, her medical journey will be uniquely her own. Our role is to assist, regardless of the outcome. It is easy to claim credit when a successful medical course is achieved. It is a far greater challenge not to abandon the patient when the outcome is less than desired. Yet in that challenge resonates the very essence of medicine. When, following a stormy medical course, the patient's family thanks the care provider for everything he or she did, even if it did not produce the desired outcome, the family is speaking from the heart. In short, the message is, "With your [the care provider's] help, we almost made it." In this setting, honesty and openness guide the discussion. It is understandable, then, why full disclosure does not differentiate harmful from harmless outcomes and thus treats them similarly.

Full disclosure in its most complete form, however, is an acknowledgment of accountability. It begins by providing to the patient and family information about the outcome and the events that led to that outcome. Having provided the facts to the family, the care provider appropriately offers condolences if an adverse outcome occurred in the absence of a care provider's ability to change the outcome. But if, armed with available medical facts, the care provider chose a management that produced the adverse outcome, this relationship of action to outcome must be addressed. Here, accountability could be paraphrased as, "With the facts I had at the time, I made the best decision I could." That statement would be followed by either, "Even knowing the outcome and with the information I had, I most likely would do the same thing again" or "Knowing the outcome, I probably would have chosen a different course of action." Here, acknowledging accountability does not impart legal blame. It simply says, "I did the best I could with the facts I had." It does differentiate outcomes affected by one's medical judgment from those unrelated to one's care plan.

What completes the process of full disclosure is a discussion of future needs. If additional medical services are needed or community resources must be identified to offer the family continued support as they negotiate the challenges of the adverse outcome, then this future-oriented discussion may carry equal weight with the disclosure of events.

Full disclosure also necessitates that programmatic issues linked to the outcome are discussed with the patient and her family as part of a root cause analysis. This risk management tool, in which the roles of each of the care providers and institution policies affecting the adverse outcome are reviewed methodically, may offer solutions to prevent future events. By bringing institutional responsibility into the discussion, the message conveyed is that future patients will be spared the adverse outcome as a result of the reevaluation of how care is provided in this circumstance.

In essence, full disclosure promotes the best qualities of medicine: honesty, integrity, and compassion.

A STRUCTURED APPROACH TO CONVERSATIONS: THE "FEARED FACTOR"

Most house staff and attendings share a sense of apprehension when they are about to engage in a conversation with a patient about an unintended adverse outcome. Few were educated in this form of communication. In fact, most would acknowledge that they never had a formal lecture in medical school or residency on the art of delivering bad news. Their skills, whatever they are, may be drawn from anecdotal cases where a more senior care provider permitted them to attend while such a conversation occurred. Fewer even, as young care providers, have experienced personal tragedy, whereby the care provider (or family member) becomes the care receiver.

The apprehension that care providers feel in anticipation of such a communication may arise from two different circumstances. First are cases in which the care provider must deliver bad news about a medical event that was not preventable. Imagine the encounter with the woman who unexpectedly is diagnosed in the ultrasound laboratory with a spontaneous fetal death, or the woman who develops severe preeclampsia and must be delivered prematurely, perhaps to the detriment of the premature newborn. In this anticipated conversation, what does the care provider fear? Perhaps it is the sense of his or her inadequacy, the inability, because of inexperience, to respond to the grief reaction, the tears, and even the outrage. What is the next sentence that should follow the statement, "Mrs. J.D., our ultrasound study has indicated that your baby [fetus] has died"? Certainly, the phrase "I am sorry" is human, shows compassion, and provides a momentary safe harbor. But what then? Does the care provider sit in silence with the patient? Does he or she leave the room briefly (to allow the patient and partner some private time), or is there the impulse simply to get out of the room as fast as possible?

What of the anxiety and apprehension felt by the care provider faced with a bad outcome who might (or should) have carried out a different therapy that would have produced a different outcome? This situation, handled improperly, offers the greatest potential for legal action. Were the patient and her family aware of the risks? Did the family misinterpret events or action plans? Or are they correct in assuming that a better plan would have produced a better outcome? And you, the care provider, were responsible.

We live in a litigious world where each person has the right to seek legal redress against his or her care provider. Some do so to cover the financial costs of short-term and long-term care following an adverse event. Of those cases, some will be dismissed as frivolous, and some will be deemed a bad outcome for which no one was at fault. But others will be attributed to the inexperience or bad judgment of the care provider.

Still other patients will sue because this avenue is their only means of reestablishing control over their lives. Whether out of anger or frustration, misinterpretation or family urging, these cases represent the product of ineffective communication. The young care provider may ask, "What good is it for me to talk to this family if my care really did result in a bad outcome? They are going to sue me anyhow." In fact, that a patient experienced an adverse outcome and that an alternative type of care might have made a difference does not inevitably mean the patient will sue. On numerous occasions when I have been asked to intervene in a discussion between care provider and patient following an adverse event, I have heard the patient say, "I'm really angry at all of you, but at least you had the courage to meet with us. We're not going to sue. We just wanted to see if you would be honest."

The young care provider next may say, "I'm afraid I will get into such a conversation and lose my way, lose track of where our discussion should go and forget the issues that should be covered." In fact, there is a simple way to structure such a conversation. We offer the acronym FEARED, an emotion felt by care providers confronted with those situations. We believe that that this sequence of statements offers such a structured approach:

> Get all the Facts.
> Express Empathy and Educate.
Search for sources of Anger.
> Have the patient Relate back to you her understanding of your explanation.
> Evaluate the Extended family response.
> Document the conversation.

Get All the Facts

A brief review of the entire case establishes a factual basis for the rest of the discussion. The clinician might say, "Mrs. J., I have reviewed your chart and hospital course and have reconstructed the events as follows . . ."

Express Empathy and Educate

An educated evaluation follows the case review. The caregiver might say something like this to the patient: "I speak for our entire group in saying how sorry we are for [the unanticipated event]. Medicine is an art form, not a mathematical equation. When bad things happen, it is our obligation to examine carefully the events to understand better if this could have been prevented, whether we should alter our practice, and, as important, explore how we can help you and your family as you move forward. My assessment of the sequence of events is . . ."

Search for Sources of Anger

This is the hardest part of the conversation, and the hardest question the caregiver can ask the patient. "Mrs. J., after such a disturbing experience, it is not unusual for some people to feel angry. Do you have those feelings, and if so, where are they directed?" The care provider's fear of asking this question comes from feeling that if the answer is, "Yes, I am angry at YOU, doctor!" he or she will lose control of the conversation. In fact, this question, phrased in the third person, may lead to a truly constructive dialogue. The real issue is what the care provider can say if the patient states that the provider was the responsible person for the bad outcome. The follow-up response to such an answer is quite important: "I am sorry you feel that way, but it is understandable. Please tell me how you arrived at that conclusion." The care provider must listen carefully for misinterpretations made by the patient or family members in the event that misconceptions represent the foundation of the anger but also offer the best opportunity to correct the facts. But what if they are correct? The initial statement in response to their anger, if based on a correct conclusion, is simply, "You may be correct that a different plan would have produced a better outcome." At this point, the care provider may have only honesty and compassion as a defense. Still, used properly, they may be sufficient to avert a lawsuit.

Have the Patient Relate Back Your Explanation

As the conversation moves toward conclusion, it is important to evaluate how well your explanations were understood. A simple question such as, "Mrs. J., it is very important that I know that you have understood my explanations and the medical issues that we have discussed. Please relate back to me your understanding of our conversation and if there are any areas that we should repeat or expand."

Evaluate the Extended Family's Understanding

At times, the inability of extended family members to understand the sequence of events leading to a bad outcome produces a slow, smoldering anger that surfaces weeks or months later. To decrease this possibility, a direct address to the family members attending such a discussion is important. The statement might be, "Many times family members feel left out when these difficult conversations are held. You all have heard our discussion. Are there issues that you feel we should cover in more depth?"

Document the Conversation

The purpose of documentation is to capture in writing the details of the meeting and the issues discussed as accurately as possible. Certain characteristics of the documentation always should be present. It should be written legibly, dated and timed, and contain the names of all of the individuals involved in the conversation and the details of the discussion. The issues addressed should be carefully described, and the questions or issues raised by the family should be documented. If the conversation occurs over several days, then at some point, a summary of the series of conversations should be entered into the record. Any laboratory data or results of other tests that apply to the discussion should be entered into the record.

Issues raised by the family are fundamental to this notation. The facts or opinions that the family volunteers may be useful to the health care organization in getting to the root cause and the family reaction to the event. It must be emphasized that factual documentation is essential for accuracy. The care provider's opinions of his or her care should not be entered into this documentation. Conjecture, fault, or blame should not be documented either.

The following information should be documented:

- The date and duration of the conference
- The names of the care provider, patient, partner (if present), and family members
- A brief description of the discussion that includes the following information:

  The facts of the case and the outcome and tone of conversation

  Sources of anger

The patient's level of understanding

Any issues raised by extended family members

Confirmation that the documentation was done immediately after the meeting

- How care providers intend to follow up with the family

CONCLUSION

The conversation to deliver and discuss bad news after an unanticipated adverse event need not be traumatic. Instead, with the proper structure, it can be turned into a compassionate, constructive dialogue. Having a conversation with a family after the successful birth of a healthy newborn is easy. Offering a conversation with a family after an adverse unanticipated event draws on the noblest resources in medicine: compassion and communication.

CHAPTER 4

Conversations to Diffuse Anger

I t is one thing to state that care providers should learn better how to converse with patients. It is quite another to provide examples of strategies for such conversations, since each medical event has its unique circumstances and each patient is unique in her reaction to those circumstances.

In this and the next two chapters, we present a series of conversations. Although none of the cases represents an actual encounter, the description of the event in each case has been drawn from a similar occurrence, and the conversation with the family has been modified to emphasize certain learning points. Each case begins with a description of a clinical event, followed by a series of questions that the care provider might consider prior to such a discussion with the patient. An overview of the case is presented, followed by basic principles, and finally how a conversation might go with the hypothetical patient and her family.

What do I say when a colleague calls and says, "I've never encountered this before, and I know I did a bad job. Please help me understand how I could have managed it differently"?

A young colleague you know only slightly calls you one evening at home, and her voice expresses distress. She says that she has just cared for her first patient with a late-gestation intrauterine demise and has managed it badly. She acknowledges that during her residency, she never had any training in talking with patients in such circumstances and therefore has no skills on which to rely.

The family of the woman she delivered is very distressed by the care she received and has written a letter to the CEO of her hospital. The CEO now demands that she meet with the family, explain why things were done poorly, and indicate to them how the care should have been provided. She relates her experience and the content of the patient's letter to the CEO to you as follows:

R.J. is a twenty-year-old Gravida 1 (G1), Para 0 (P0), with an uncomplicated prenatal course until thirty-nine weeks' gestation. R.J. had telephoned my office the evening before to make an appointment because she hadn't felt the baby move through the afternoon. She was given an appointment to see me the next afternoon. When she was seen in the office, R.J.'s vital signs were stable, but no fetal heart tones were found. R.J. was sent home with instructions to make an appointment at the local ultrasound-radiology center for the next day to evaluate these findings further.

R.J. arrived at the ultrasound radiology center at the appointed time. After checking in with the receptionist, she sat in a waiting room with other patients, including several pregnant women scheduled for ultrasounds. After a lengthy wait, she was ushered into an ultrasound room. The sonographer scanned R.J. quickly, then departed without a word. A few minutes later, the radiologist entered the room and performed a second equally brief scan. The machine was turned off, and R.J. was sent home with the radiologist's comment, "The ultrasound report will be sent to your doctor."

The next morning, R.J. returned to my obstetric office, confused and concerned. Again, she sat in a waiting room with several pregnant women. Finally, she was brought into an examination room, where I told her that "the ultrasound report indicates that there is no fetal cardiac activity." Unclear as to exactly what had occurred, R.J. asked if her baby was "all right." I then told her that her baby was dead and induction of labor would be necessary.

I began a lengthy explanation about causes of fetal death, tests, and follow-up, but R.J., apparently stunned by the news, interrupted the conversation. She stated that she wanted to go home to be with her family that night and asked to be induced in the morning. Since she had come to the office alone, she drove home with difficulty and later told me she remembered few details of how or when she got there.

The next morning, R.J. was admitted to a labor room that was occupied by another pregnant woman who was on a fetal monitor. R.J.'s Pitocin induction was begun, resulting in rapid progression of labor and spontaneous delivery of a macerated male fetus. Later, the baby's autopsy report revealed that the death had occurred several days before R.J. was seen in the office. At delivery, I placed the stillborn boy into a pan, which then was placed on the delivery cart and removed from the room. When R.J. asked whether she had had a boy or a girl, a nurse responded, "We don't know." Immediately postpartum, while R.J. and her husband were in a fully occupied six-bed recovery room, uterine bleeding was noted and Hemobate, uterine massage, and Pitocin were used to provide hemostasis.

Once R.J. was back in her semiprivate room, she and her husband were permitted to hold their baby son. Spontaneously, R.J. experienced enormous relief: "My baby is normal! I thought that the doctors couldn't tell if he was a boy or a girl." Then she asked the nurse to take a photograph of her son. The nurse, appalled by the baby's appearance, took the dead fetus to a dimly lighted room and used the instant camera from labor and delivery to snap a quick picture of the baby lying flat on a blanket. She covered most of the baby's body with a blanket, believing that the family would be saddened to see the skin discoloration and desquamation that death had produced in the baby. Shortly after, the nurse came back into the room and told the family, "It is the ward rule that after a baby dies, the family can stay with the baby for twenty minutes. It is time for the baby to be taken to the morgue."

A while later, R.J. was asked if the family wanted an autopsy performed. When she and her husband indicated a reluctance, her nurse supported the decision by commenting that seldom in her experience did autopsy results offer any important information as to cause of death.

Later that afternoon, I dropped by and reinforced R.J. and her husband's decision by commenting that an autopsy would make any type of open casket at a funeral impossible. R.J. kept referring to her stillborn as "John," something I kept forgetting in our conversation. After all, the stillborn had been dead for several days. I focused my comments on R.J.'s postpartum bleeding and described in detail the types of medication used to decrease the bleeding. I stated that, unfortunately, my need to round on several other patients prevented me from conducting a lengthier discussion about R.J.'s son's death. I commented that perhaps at her six-week postpartum visit, we could go into this in more detail. As I prepared to leave, I mentioned that because of the degree of skin changes exhibited by their baby, cremation may be a preferred route to burial. I commented also that if they chose to have the cremation done at the hospital, I was sure that they would be able to obtain their baby's ashes. After all, private funeral homes providing cremation offer such services. R.J. and her husband took in my suggestions and asked one more favor: Could their son be circumcised? I was visibly taken aback and politely denied their request, indicating that I would not want that done if this were my son. At the last minute, R.J. changed her mind about the autopsy. She and her husband signed the permission forms.

The next morning, R.J. was discharged home, having been given a six-week appointment for a postpartum physical examination and Pap smear, as well as brief instructions about birth control. When R.J. indicated to her nurse that she was experiencing breast engorgement, her nurse stated, "It will go away. You are not going to need it anyhow." R.J. and her husband also were advised not to engage in sexual intercourse "until I said it was okay again." As R.J. and her husband were escorted downstairs to the discharge area, another postpartum patient holding her newborn sat in a wheelchair next to that of R.J., while both husbands departed to bring the cars to the patient-discharge area.

Three weeks after the discharge, the family sent a letter to the CEO of the hospital expressing their appreciation for the care provided by the nurses and the compassion shown by the housekeepers but their outrage toward me as their physician, particularly after they asked neighbors and friends about the care they should have expected. They demanded to meet with me.

Questions that kept running through my mind were:

- When should R.J. have been seen in the office after she called the first time?
- When should the ultrasound have been performed?
- How should she have been treated at the radiology center?
- Should the ultrasound scan have been performed differently?
- When should I have seen her after the ultrasound scan?
- How should the news have been given to R.J.?
- Should I have let her drive home alone?
- Should I have managed her labor and delivery differently?
- Should she have been placed in a private room?
- How does one take a picture of a dead baby?
- Should all parents of a stillborn be encouraged to have an autopsy?
- Were my statements about autopsy, cremation, and an open casket correct?
- Should the family have been allowed more time with their dead son?
- Should I have agreed to a circumcision?
- Should I have made more time to spend with R.J. while she was in the hospital?
- How should the issue of breast engorgement have been managed?
- When should I have seen her first in the postpartum period?
- What questions could I ask at that first outpatient visit?
- Could R.J.'s departure from the hospital have been done more sensitively?

This hypothetical case illustrates the errors that well-intended care providers make in their management of a patient with a pregnancy loss. The errors began when the patient, having telephoned regarding a decrease in fetal movement, had to wait until the next afternoon. The care in the radiology center was superficial, and asking the patient to sit in a general waiting room with other patients shows that the care providers were not providing R.J. individualized care but simply routine care. That R.J. was not referred immediately back to her care provider following the ultrasound scan compounded the mistakes, as did the imprecise manner in which the information regarding her baby's death was given to her in the office. Providing a lengthy explanation of the possible causes of death when a patient at best can absorb only a brief description of the findings is inappropriate, and allowing her to drive home alone after receiving this information is dangerous.

In labor and delivery, placing the delivered stillborn son into a pan was careless and insensitive. That mental image may be seared in the minds of the woman and her attending family members forever. Perhaps the care provider was uncomfortable handling a dead baby. That should not be an excuse. Delivering the baby into a blanket that then is carefully wrapped around the body is an appropriate and gracious gesture. Postpartum, placing the woman in a fully occupied recovery room exacerbated the problem, as did the insensitive way in which the nurse reacted to R.J.'s request to have a picture taken of her baby. The care provider's response to the autopsy showed a lack of understanding of its importance. The fact that nearly a quarter of autopsies result in a change or alteration of the final diagnosis underscores their value for subsequent counseling. The physician indicated that she did not have adequate time on rounds to sit with the patient. That was an error in judgment, since this is the best opportunity to begin a discussion that can be continued in the outpatient setting. Not knowing the hospital policies for cremation was inexcusable, as was the reaction to the parents' request for circumcision. That the nurse legislated a brief interval for the family to visit with their baby before he was moved to the morgue was inappropriate, as was the nurse's response to R.J.'s concerns about breast engorgement. Clearly no lactation consultation was requested by the care provider to explain to R.J. the sad process of breast engorgement after a baby dies.

There was no effort in this hypothetical case to engage a social worker or member of the patient's or hospital clergy in her inpatient care. Two valued members of the health team, her primary care physician and the intended pediatrician for this newborn, were not notified. That the nurses

What Do I Say?

and the housekeeper were complimented in the letter to the CEO for their attentiveness demonstrates the simple principle that all professionals in the health care environment can learn the universal language of compassion. From physicians to housekeepers, the expression, "I am sorry that your baby died," will be remembered long after the individual events of the hospitalization begin to blur.

Giving R.J. a six-week postpartum appointment was an error; the first outpatient visit should occur within the first week to ten days after discharge. It is no surprise that on discharge, R.J. felt abandoned by her health community, thus prompting an angry letter to the CEO.

How could this have been done better? R.J. should have been seen that evening when she first called her obstetrician about decreased fetal movement. The finding that the baby had died several days before does not excuse this error in response. Any woman who calls her obstetrician with a perception of decreased fetal movement should be seen and evaluated immediately. At the radiology center, the receptionist should have been forewarned that the patient was coming so that R.J. could be ushered into a separate room and not left in the general waiting area. The ultrasound scan should have been conducted over several minutes, thereby communicating to R.J. that a complete examination was carried out. The comment that the ultrasound report would be sent to her doctor when in fact R.J. was fearful of the possibility that her baby had died should instead either have been a statement of the actual findings, or, "I am sending the report to your doctor immediately and will call him [or her] now to seek advice as to whether you should go to the office for a further discussion of the findings." Unfortunately, even this information conveys the message that the findings were not normal and that everything is not fine.

When R.J. returned to her obstetrician's office, she should have been ushered into a private room and given the information briefly but clearly. The obstetrician should have formulated a brief script to present to the patient explaining that her baby had died. No lengthy discussion should have occurred at that time. R.J. should have been encouraged to call a family member to come and drive her home instead of allowing her to drive home alone.

When R.J. was admitted into the hospital for induction of labor, she should have been placed in a private room. If R.J.'s health plan balked at this idea, a telephone call could have been made to gain approval for this step. The baby should have been delivered with care into a blanket so that the parents could hold their baby. Providing a description of the baby to the parents immediately after delivery, pointing out some of the normal features, reduces the fears that the baby was grotesque. Emphasizing the positive features or characteristics of their baby captures a mental image for parents to remember.

The nurse should have taken more time to take photographs of the baby and used a 35 mm or digital camera. Simple techniques make for a better picture, such as turning the head to exhibit the baby's jaw line or forehead, or determining whether the baby's mouth or eyes should be open. For taking pictures of babies with malformations, placing a blanket over those aspects of the baby's body that are malformed provides a more normal-appearing photograph. Many parents, however, want a picture of their fully exposed baby. This photograph also should be taken. In fact, several pictures should be taken so that the parents can choose which ones they prefer. For parents who decline a photograph, suggest that with their permission, several will be taken and placed on file if they want them at a later date. Be sensitive to ethnic and religious customs. For some cultures, picture taking is not appropriate.

An autopsy should have been encouraged. For many parents, a normal autopsy result is reassuring, even if the outcome was not the desired one. If the autopsy reveals findings that were not anticipated, this information may be important in counseling for future pregnancies and in providing the answer to the question, "Why did this happen to us?"

While R.J. was in the hospital, the physician should have rounded on her twice daily and should have taken the time to meet with her (and the family if R.J. so desired) at least once to conduct a more thorough conversation about the diagnosis, management, and follow-up. (The ten-minute chat is helpful. See page 157.) Simple questions such as, "How are you feeling?" and "What are you thinking about?" and a simple statement of condolence, "I am so sorry about your loss," likely will initiate a conversation that leads to further discussions when R.J. is next seen in the office. In these encounters, *always* use the baby's name and refrain from the phrase *the baby*. A name imparts a personality. A family name provides a bridge to the stillborn son.

All care providers should be familiar with policies for hospital cremation compared to cremation carried out by a private funeral home. Most hospitals will not give back individual ashes if cremation is performed there, whereas private funeral homes provide such services. Also, many hospitals require an autopsy if they will be performing the cremation. An autopsy does not negate an open casket at a funeral home. Autopsies now can be performed through small incisions or even as biopsies to retain the general physical appearance of the baby. One must, however, take into account cultural and religious preferences when requesting an autopsy. The following opinions were drawn from pediatric pathologists on a listserv regarding attitudes regarding autopsy:

- Among Malays who are Muslim, an autopsy is seldom requested because of religious attitudes. The placenta is buried with the body.

- The Chinese view bringing a dead baby into the household as bad luck. Many babies who die in the neonatal period are left in the hospital for disposal.

- In Ireland, the tradition is a rapid funeral within the first twenty-four to forty-eight hours following death.

- Among indigenous populations, such as aboriginals, Maoris, and Native Americans, postmortem autopsy evaluations are seldom requested.

- Among the Yanomami tribe in the Brazilian Amazon, no procedures are carried out on a deceased child. The child is cremated, and the family drinks a mixture of the ashes in a sacred beverage.

- Muslim children of North African origin do not undergo a postmortem examination when delivered in France. In contrast, Algerian pathologists do perform postmortems in Algeria on Muslim children. It is unclear whether these differences represent culture and religion.

Conversations to Diffuse Anger

- In Pakistan, no autopsies are carried out on newborns delivered in a hospital. Autopsies are encouraged for accidents and murders.

- A common belief in Hong Kong is that the body of the dead should not be disturbed; nevertheless, pediatricians encourage an autopsy for still-born fetuses and following neonatal death.

- Among some Jews (mostly Orthodox), autopsies are not sought unless there is knowledge that the findings will help another sick individual. The autopsy is restricted in scope, and the organs are returned to the body.

Requests by parents of stillborn babies for types of care usually provided to healthy newborns should not be dismissed as inappropriate. In this example, the obstetrician should have performed the circumcision. There are few rules when a baby dies. The more flexible the care provider is under these circumstances, the better the family will perceive the care that they received.

Saying goodbye to a dead baby is a gesture families carry out in unique and individual ways. No care provider or hospital staff member should compromise this privilege. A family should be allowed to stay with their stillborn baby as long as they wish. Some families prefer to spend the night with the baby before he or she is taken to the morgue. When the nurse insisted that twenty minutes was enough time, her statement was inappropriate.

When R.J. raised her concerns about breast engorgement, she should have been counseled sensitively by a lactation consultant. The grief of a baby lost is amplified by physiological events that accompany such a delivery.

Upon discharge from the hospital, R.J. should have been given an appointment to be seen in the office in the first week or ten days. Having her primary inpatient nurse call her at home the next day offers a transition into the outpatient care and counseling she will need. At that first office visit, the discussion should focus on how she was treated in the hospital, how it was to go home, and what kind of support existed at home. Other questions would be whether they had prepared a nursery and, if so, how the family was reacting to it, and what some of the questions were that the family asked the patient during that week. Other topics include advice on how to respond to friends or acquaintances unaware of the death, how men and women respond to grief, and how long the grieving process will go on. Waiting until six weeks for the first outpatient postpartum visit likely will motivate the patient to transfer to another obstetric practice.

Finally, a nurse should have escorted R.J. to the discharge area in order to avoid encounters with other women leaving with healthy babies.

Basic Principles

- Respond immediately when the patient calls because her baby is not moving.
- Evaluate the patient immediately in an ultrasound laboratory or the triage area.
- Notify the ultrasound unit or labor and delivery unit if the patient is coming because of a lack of fetal movement.
- The radiologist or perinatologist performing the scan of a patient whose baby may have died should conduct a complete scan, even if the diagnosis of fetal death is evident.
- The radiologist or perinatologist should notify the patient's physician immediately about the scan findings if they are bad.
- The patient should go to the care provider's office immediately.
- The bad news should be given briefly but clearly.
- Inquire about means of transportation home.
- In labor and delivery, place the patient in a private room.
- Deliver the baby in a sensitive manner.
- Have the patient recover in a private room.
- Recognize the value of pictures of the baby and an autopsy.
- Respect the requests of parents for special treatment of their baby, even if the request seems unusual.
- Allow the family as much time with their baby as they need.
- Prepare the patient for the emotional conflict of breast engorgement after a pregnancy lost.

- Discuss strategies for coping once the woman and partner return home.
- Have the patient seen in the office in the first week postpartum.
- Notify her primary care provider and pediatrician of the adverse event.

Here is how the conversation might go three weeks after discharge in the doctor's office when R.J. and her family are invited so that you can respond to their feelings of hurt and anger regarding their care.

Points to Cover	The Conversation
Be courteous.	R.J., I thank you and your family for coming to the office to provide us the opportunity to discuss the events that occurred in the hospital and for me to be able to answer questions that you have. From my analysis of your care, I believe there were many aspects of your care that should have been done differently to convey to you our respect for you and John.
Respond immediately.	The night you called because you did not feel your baby moving, we should have seen you to evaluate your baby.
Call ahead.	If that meant sending you to a radiology or perinatal unit, we should have called the receptionist at the unit so that you could have been brought into a separate room and not forced to sit with other pregnant women.
Call for the results immediately; then see the patient.	When the scan was over, the radiologist should have called me immediately with the results, and I then should have had you come to my office.
Be concise.	When I gave you the news, I should have given it briefly and concisely. I should have given you some private time, and then I should have asked if you had any questions.

Points to Cover	The Conversation
Ask about transportation.	I also should have inquired as to whether you had transportation home or whether a family member could come to pick you up.
Show compassion.	In labor and delivery, we should have put you in a private room and when your son, John, delivered, I should have wrapped him in a blanket so that you could hold him.
Pictures in the postpartum period.	When you requested it, we should have taken several thoughtful pictures of John, some with your son partially covered to give a more normal appearance and some fully exposed. Later, you could select the pictures you wanted.
The autopsy.	We should have encouraged you to agree to an autopsy because a significant number of autopsies lead to a change in the diagnosis. Also, we should have recognized that if the autopsy was normal, this information would have given you some reassurance.
Cremation.	We have since checked on the hospital policy for cremation and now teach other care providers that ashes are not available when the hospital carries out the cremation. This is different than when cremation is carried out by a private funeral home. Moreover, we know that even if an autopsy had been done, an open casket could have been requested.
Find time to talk.	I should have spent more time with you in the hospital, finding at least one period between rounds where we could meet together with your family to discuss the death of your son.

Points to Cover	The Conversation
Be flexible.	When you asked that John be circumcised, I should have willingly agreed to perform that without questioning whether I would have selected that choice myself. We should have allowed you as much time with John as you wanted before he was taken to the morgue and not imposed on you our own time limits.
Breast engorgement.	When you described breast engorgement to your nurse, we should have had a lactation consultant help you through this difficult physiological event.
Leaving the hospital.	I then should have had you escorted to your car by one of our nurses to offer you some privacy on your way home.
Notify appropriate caregivers and pediatrician.	I should have called your primary care physician and pediatrician to provide them the information on John's death.
First postpartum visit.	I should have seen you in my office in the first week after discharge to review the hospital care and to seek questions that you had regarding your son's death.
A letter.	During that visit, I might have suggested several strategies that could have helped you. For instance, I would have suggested that you write your thoughts about John on paper. You even might have developed this as a letter to your son. These types of letters capture the deepest emotions that are felt at the time and are difficult to recreate weeks or months later.

Points to Cover	The Conversation
Offer solutions.	I should have inquired as to whether you had set up a nursery and what happened to it when you knew John had died. Was it dismantled, did you close it off from the rest of the house, or did it offer you peace that you loved your son so much? I also should have suggested that you prepare some simple answers as responses to questions that friends or acquaintances might ask at inappropriate times, such as chance meetings at your local grocery store or cleaners when they first see you and yet do not know about your pregnancy loss.
Advice on long-term recovery: Men versus women.	I would have told you that you and your husband will recover from this terrible loss successfully but at different rates. Some days, you will be feeling more energy, and he will not. Other times, the reverse will be true. Also, men tend to recover differently than women do from such a tragedy. Men will fill their time with activity and may not want to discuss the baby's death. They likely will not be asked by their male coworkers about it either. Women, in contrast, tend to think about it much more, discuss it in more depth with other women, and take longer to work through the pain and grief.
Follow-up.	Finally, I should have arranged for us to meet again within one or two weeks after your discharge to continue our discussion as to why we believe your baby died. When the final autopsy report is available, we should sit down to review it and how you are recovering.

Points to Cover	The Conversation
Apology.	The gestures that I have mentioned that should have been done differently unfortunately would not have changed the outcome for your baby. They would, however, have made your experience less painful.
Document.	[A thorough documentation of the discussion should be entered into the medical record.]

What do I say to the family when a disagreement on management between a doctor and nurse occurred in front of the patient and was accompanied by a bad outcome?

J.P., a twenty-two-year-old G1, P0 from a large, closely knit family, is admitted to your labor and delivery suite at forty weeks' gestation in early labor. You are covering labor and delivery for your group during the day, but have scheduled several appointments for patients in your office this evening. J.P.'s labor advances slowly, and you choose to augment her with Pitocin. You present this to J.P. and her family when her nurse, B.A., indicates to you that she would like to have a private conversation about her concerns regarding the fetal heart rate tracing. B.A. and you step out of the room. B.A. states that she has noticed episodes in the fetal heart rate tracing that are not very reassuring. Because you have several patients in labor, you brush off these comments by B.A. and write the orders for Pitocin.

Within the hour, B.A. calls you into the room to look at the fetal heart rate tracing. There now are variable decelerations and some decrease in heart rate variability. B.A. suggests that the Pitocin be turned off. You motion B.A. to the end of the room, where you think you are out of hearing range of the family, and say, "Look, you don't understand these things. I am the doctor, and I am in charge. I want you to push the Pitocin until the baby cannot tolerate it. Then we will do a cesarean section, and I will get to my office on time to see patients."

You leave the room and later are told that family members clearly heard that discussion. Picture the dilemma of the nurse who now must turn back toward the patient following that confrontational discussion. Four options are available to her:

- Return to the bedside, but through silence, express her feelings of discomfort at the commands she has received from the physician. It is not likely that the patient will miss this body language.
- Return to the bedside, but under her breath chastise the physician for ordering her to proceed with the Pitocin. Her actions in this more aggressive approach may seek a personal victory in this doctor-nurse debate, but it will be short-lived. The patient need not read body language to understand the conflict into which she now has been placed as a result of the dispute by the two care providers.
- Refuse to proceed with the management plan as dictated by the physician. How does the nurse avoid being accused of abandoning the patient while at the same time recognizing that in many hospital settings, this refusal may jeopardize her job?
- Search for a compromise to this overheard confrontation by explaining to the patient that the discussion brings out both sides of the issue. Returning to the bedside, the nurse may say to the patient, "You obviously overhead our discussion about your management. When two well-trained professionals disagree on a medical care plan, this disagreement often leads to improved care by bringing together the backgrounds and experiences of each care provider. In your case, the physician has asked that I increase the Pitocin. We will do this slowly and keep a vigilance for your baby's health in case there are any signs that your baby is not tolerating the labor."

B.A. acquiesces to your commands, and the Pitocin is increased. Within thirty minutes, the fetal heart rate tracing suddenly exhibits an abrupt deceleration and a stat cesarean section is performed, productive of a 3200-gram newborn male with one-, five-, and ten-minute Apgar scores of 1, 1, 3 and cord blood gas values indicating significant metabolic acidosis. The pediatrician carries out a full resuscitation, and the newborn is moved quickly to the neonatal intensive care nursery (NICU). The newborn male exhibits seizures in the NICU and requires transfer to the regional perinatal center along with his mother. The baby has a stormy course, ultimately controlled by phenobarbital but later will show developmental disorders.

The next morning, your medical director informs you that you and B.A. will report to his office at noon to explain your actions: the family already has talked to him about initiating a lawsuit based on the conversations they overheard. They specifically refer to the dispute you and B.A. had regarding interpretation of the fetal heart retracing and the subsequent Pitocin management.

As you wait outside the office of the medical director, many thoughts race through your mind:

- Where should a discussion occur between a doctor and nurse when there is a differing opinion regarding care?
- If there is no resolution, how should a chain of command be used to resolve this difference of opinion in management?
- How should the events leading up to the cesarean section be presented to this family?
- What format should be used to present this information?

This unprofessional interaction between physician and nurse is not unique to obstetrics; it applies to other fields of medicine as well. Three issues must be addressed:

- What are the facts?
- How does a medical professional use the chain of command appropriately to take issues to a higher level when the care being provided is not consistent with his or her opinion of appropriate management?
- How is this information then conveyed to the family who witnessed this unprofessional interaction that was followed by this adverse event?

The first step for the medical director is to bring together the chairperson of obstetrics and gynecology, the chief of obstetric nursing, and each of the medical professionals who were involved in the care of J.P. This closed session allows a full disclosure of the events and the communications surrounding those events. To the extent permitted under applicable state law and health facility policy, this meeting should be considered a peer review conference or confidential closed quality assurance meeting, and the information generated should be kept in a confidential file after the facts have been discussed.

In the meeting, the proper use of chain of command should be reviewed. Use of the chain of command provides protection to care providers but also guidance when they find themselves caught in a dispute over the management of a patient's care. When a difference of opinion on management occurred between physician and nurse, that discussion should have been taken outside the patient's room to an area of privacy. Understandably, some medical decisions will be controversial. Each party is owed the professional right to make his or her case.

Historically, the obstetrician was considered the captain of the ship. The idea was that the physician was responsible for the management of the patient's care. Although nursing staff and others were employed by the hospital, they were acting under the direction or control of the physician—hence, the idea of likening the physician to the captain of the ship. Unfortunately, when problems occurred and lawsuits resulted, many doctors were hesitant to take on the mantle of captain. The law has made it clear that a hospital has a responsibility to oversee or provide for quality patient care. If nurses failed to alert hospital officials about patient care issues and, as a reasonably foreseeable result, harm ensued, accountability could be imputed to the hospital through the errors and omissions of nurse-employees. Moreover, the law has come to recognize that in today's medical environment, the care provided a patient represents the collective efforts of a team of care providers. In this case, the doctor and nurse disagreed over the interpretation of the fetal heart rate tracing. A private discussion in another room would have allowed each to express his or her concerns. That interchange alone should have produced an appropriate management plan. In this case, it did not. It is for this very situation that a chain-of-command policy exists.

Each professional has his or her own chain of command when such a conflict exists. The physician may seek the advice of a colleague. The nurse has a nurse leader or charge nurse above him or her and a nursing director above that individual. The chairperson of the department and chief of obstetric nursing are responsible for all care provided in the obstetrics unit, and the medical director and hospital director of nursing carry the responsibility of medical care for the institution. This chain of command rarely is needed, but it becomes essential if one of the care providers participating in J.P.'s care cannot in good conscience remain involved if the care is perceived as inappropriate or, worse, dangerous.

Once the facts have been gathered and a chain of command has been identified, the next question is how to approach the family and who should be involved. If the conflict between doctor and nurse has been resolved, then the two may wish to meet with the family in order to discuss the management. Otherwise, the medical director may instruct the chief of the department of obstetrics and gynecology as arbitrator to conduct this discussion since he or she may be more familiar with the case and also has an obstetrics background. The key point is not to exacerbate the problem but instead to provide an honest description of the differences of opinion that the family overheard. It is possible that the outcome of the sudden fetal bradycardia was not a result of the Pitocin administration. If that were the case, it should be stated. Nonetheless, the family heard this discussion and the inappropriate statement that "pushing the Pitocin might shorten the labor" leading to a cesarean section so that the doctor could get to his office that evening. In this theoretical case, it may be necessary for the physician to admit openly that his comments were inappropriate and to apologize for such comments, even if the action did not produce the final event. A plan for ongoing care for both the mother and the newborn should be presented, and further meetings with the family should be scheduled to reduce their anger and suspicion.

Basic Principles

- Gather all care providers together for a fact-finding conference, and document the facts.

- Recognize the importance of a chain-of-command policy for both the physician and nurse, and identify the key individuals at each level of the chain of command.

- Arrange to meet with the family to discuss the care that J.P. received.

- Have the nurse and physician meet with the family, if appropriate, or the physician alone should be there. If necessary, the chairperson of the department or the medical director may need to serve as mediator.

- Acknowledge the dispute in management, and seek the reaction of the family to this dispute.

- Inquire about anger felt by the family.

- Inquire as to whether any extended family members have questions regarding the care.

- Develop a plan for the future care of the mother and baby.

- Document the conversation with the family, the facts, and the reaction of the family.

Here is how the actual conversation might go at the quality assurance meeting in accordance with the hospital bylaws:

Points to Cover	The Conversation
State the reason for the meeting.	As medical director, I brought you together to seek the facts regarding this case and the dispute that the family overheard.

Points to Cover	The Conversation
Case presentations.	[The doctor and nurse present their side of the argument and their interpretation of the care. They may offer their emotional reaction to this dispute and how it affected the overall management of the situation.]
Private discussions.	I am sure that you know how important it is for patients to understand how professionals work together in complicated medical care. When a dispute occurs, that dispute should be taken to a private area where both sides can be presented. That dispute never should be presented within hearing distance of the family, and neither side should ever convey to the family his or her lack of support for such management. These debates over management should be done in a private place away from the patient.
Strategy for family meeting.	[The medical director may delegate to the physician or to the physician and nurse the need to meet with the family in order to explain the differences of opinion and the clinical course that led to the outcome.] I expect that you will have this meeting with the family within the next few days, and I would like a written report of how that conversation went.
Be open.	[The meeting with the family is held the next day. The conversation might go as follows:] J.P., I appreciate the fact that you and your family have agreed to meet with me and nurse B.A. to discuss the care that you received. As you know, we did not agree on the interpretation of the fetal heart rate tracing. In retrospect, that conversation should have taken place in a private area.

Points to Cover	The Conversation
Value of professional debate.	If there is any value in debate, it is that two professionals with extensive training are putting their thoughts together to provide you the best care.
If appropriate, apologize.	It was very shortsighted of me to make an ill-advised comment about hurrying your labor so that if a cesarean section were needed, I could get back to the office. For that comment, I apologize.
Address the association of the debate to the outcome.	In reviewing the fetal heart rate tracing, I do not think the increased Pitocin had any effect on your baby's sudden bradycardia. We have sent the placenta to the pathologist for inspection and to understand why the event occurred. We want to work closely with you and your baby to make sure that the best care is given, and we hope the outcome will be good. I wish to repeat that it was inappropriate for the two of us to disagree publicly over your care, and I hope you will accept our apology.
Chain of command.	When two professionals disagree, we do have a chain of command. That chain of command allows me to seek additional information from a colleague or for your nurse to seek input from the charge nurse or even the nursing chief when significant differences of opinion arise regarding your care. I do not believe that we used that chain of command successfully and have reaffirmed this process with physicians and nurses in our department. [The conversation continues with the family members' voicing their reactions to the

Points to Cover	The Conversation
Chain of command. (cont.)	event. The meeting then is concluded.] Thank you for your time. Please call me if you have other questions. [As the family departs, they express their satisfaction with the detail and honesty expressed in the conversation.]
Document.	[A thorough documentation of the discussion is entered into the medical record.]

What do I say when a patient's interpretation of a poorly managed case is correct?

J.L. is a thirty-five-year-old G1, P0 who is seen in your triage area by one of your partners. She is at thirty-nine weeks' gestation and complaining of irregular uterine contractions. On examination, the patient is found to be 5 centimeters dilated with the fetal head at a −2 station. The patient is observed on your labor deck for approximately two hours and during that period experiences a decrease in uterine activity; during the third hour, she feels no more uterine contractions at all. Your partner elects to discharge her home with instructions that when uterine activity begins again, to return to the labor and delivery triage area. The patient returns home and during the night experiences no more uterine activity.

The next morning, upon awakening, she notices decreased fetal movement and then the absence of fetal activity. Understandably anxious, she presents to triage, and there are no fetal heart tones noted. The family grieves appropriately as you develop a plan for induction of labor. Labor is rapid, and the female stillborn is delivered without complications. No visible explanation for the intrauterine fetal demise can be drawn from the physical inspection of the fetus.

That afternoon, as you make rounds on your patient, she expresses extreme grief but also intense anger that she was sent home. She attributes this decision as the explanation for her baby's death.

You ask yourself:

- How honest should I be?
- Should I admit it if I disagree with the care she received?
- How can I deflect her anger?
- Can any good come out of this bad outcome?

This is a dilemma that frequently is encountered in obstetrics. As groups become larger and cross-coverage becomes the normal scheduling setup, management often is carried out by one's partner or even a member of another group who is providing cross-coverage. The principles that apply here rest on allowing ample time to discuss this case with the family, being honest, and being willing to provide your own opinion. You also may need to respond to the question whether an alternative management (and different outcome) would have been preferable or whether the outcome was independent of either of these two decisions. Finally, the conversation must be constructed to diffuse anger and clarify the issues. It is essential that the care provider determine in the discussion if this anger is focused indirectly at either family dynamics or external issues that restricted the ability of the patient to seek obstetric care.

Basic Principles

- Be honest.
- Diffuse anger. Is the anger directed at the right issue?
- Provide an opinion if an alternative management should have been applied.
- If appropriate, suggest that lessons learned from this event may be applied to help someone in the future.
- Document the discussion.

Here is how the actual conversation might go:

Points to Cover	The Conversation
Introduction.	Mrs. L., I appreciate the fact that you and your family were able to come into my office today to discuss the death of your baby daughter. We recognize that this is a very sad time and that it must have been very difficult for you to come into the office, since this visit undoubtedly brings up a lot of uncomfortable feelings.
Define the timetable for the conversation.	I have rearranged my schedule for the afternoon and therefore am able to spend as much time with you and your family as needed to answer questions and review the events that occurred.
The facts.	As I understand them, the events are as follows. [A full disclosure of the facts of the case is presented in an unemotional way, but in a manner that does not indicate any kind of judgmental opinions or obscure any of the facts.]
Search for anger.	Mrs. L., many family members find at a moment like this that they not only are overwhelmed with grief, but they also have strong feelings of anger. Are these the types of feelings that you have had?
Divergent pathways of response; be prepared for direct questions of accountability.	[At this point, one of two reactions may be encountered. The family may acknowledge that they do not perceive that any mismanagement occurred; they are only seeking information so that they can better understand how such a tragedy could have occurred. But under the circumstances of this particular case, it would be understandable if the family lashed out at the care provider while expressing great anger and even the possibility of legal action. They also may directly ask the care provider whether this type of management would have occurred under his or her call. Honesty at this point is fundamental in establishing a base for further discussion.]

Points to Cover	The Conversation
Discuss management protocols.	Mrs. L., I can understand that you might be very angry and wonder whether, in fact, it was appropriate that you were sent home when you were 5 centimeters dilated at this late stage of pregnancy. It is simplistic for me to pass judgment on that decision because in retrospect, we know that the outcome was bad. In medicine, there often are different ways to approach a problem. Some care providers might have sent you home, realizing that they did not want to inconvenience you by a prolonged hospitalization if in fact you were not in labor. Others would have induced your labor to complete the process, realizing that you were already 5 centimeters dilated, even though your contractions had ceased.
Provide an opinion if appropriate.	I probably would have been inclined to do the latter. Nonetheless, I can understand why someone might have chosen the former, and if you had had a successful delivery, we would not be discussing these two types of management of your case.
Search for sources of anger or guilt.	[The care provider then might seek again to identify whether other sources of anger exist. For instance, when the patient went home but then perceived a decrease in fetal movement, did she have a difficult time getting someone to take her into the hospital, thereby prolonging the period in which she perceived this decrease in fetal movement? Does she herself feel that she was not acting in a timely way in returning to the hospital after there was decreased fetal movement? These questions shift

Points to Cover	The Conversation
Search for sources of anger or guilt. (cont.)	the focus from the care provider's responsibilities to that of the individual, and this shift must be done carefully. Otherwise, it may be perceived as confrontational and inappropriately redirecting the responsibility to that of the patient, as opposed to the care provider.]
Programmatic change.	[The care provider may wish to engage in a discussion of programmatic changes that the patient's bad outcome has prompted. This approach conveys to the patient that the bad outcome that she encountered possibly will lead to changes in practice that might prevent a similar occurrence in the future for another patient or another family. A discussion might include a review of the case in a management conference in which her specific care was discussed. Guidelines in the department may be reviewed in an effort to determine if lessons learned from this bad outcome could influence care for future patients. The fact that someone's baby died is a tragedy. The knowledge that one's baby's death may contribute toward improved care in the future may offer some balance in this otherwise very challenging discussion. A cautionary note: Lessons learned or programmatic change that comes as a result of an adverse event should not be stated to the patient in such a way as to suggest blame or fault.]
Document.	[A thorough documentation of the discussion should be entered into the medical record.]

How should I respond when a patient or family member directs his or her anger at me for a bad outcome that I may have been responsible for?

J.L. is a twenty-two-year-old G1 P0 with an undocumented history of low-grade hypertension. Prior to her pregnancy, she had been on various antihypertensive medications, but states that in the early part of this pregnancy, while on no medication, her blood pressure was in the normal range. She transferred into your practice late in pregnancy, and there is no evidence from her clinical course that she is indeed hypertensive. Fetal growth on ultrasound is at the twentieth percentile at thirty-four weeks' gestation and at thirty-six weeks' gestation remains at approximately that percentile. Her blood pressure at this time, however, has risen slightly, to approximately 140/88 mmHg.

In the office, she asks whether she should be on an antihypertensive medication and whether fetal monitoring in the form of a nonstress test should be initiated. You are impressed by her awareness of pregnancy risks and methods for fetal assessment, but learn that she has derived this knowledge from the Internet. You comment to her that there is no evidence that treatment of mild blood pressure elevation has an impact on care, but that she will be followed weekly and, if necessary, placed on antihypertensive medications. Moreover, fetal surveillance will be initiated if there are any additional changes in her blood pressure.

She calls you three days later, not feeling any fetal movement. On admission, there is no fetal heartbeat, and a diagnosis of intrauterine fetal death is made. At that point, her blood pressure is noted to be 160/105 mmHg and shortly after admission requires antihypertensive medication to bring it under control. Labor is initiated, but the atmosphere is tense, and the anger expressed by her family is palpable. Delivery occurs uneventfully, but on delivery of the placenta, a 50 percent placental abruption is noted. You schedule a meeting of the family in her postpartum room for that afternoon to address her anger and the unfortunate events that occurred.

You then ask yourself:

- How do I show my concern?
- Can I say "I'm sorry" without saying "I made a mistake"?
- How can I diffuse my patient's anger?
- How do I keep a calm tone through our discussion?

In this situation, like many others in obstetrics, the conversation to address the adverse outcome with the family must walk a fine line between presumed innocence and presumed guilt at the hands of the care provider. In this scenario, the patient raised concerns about the possibility of needing antihypertensive medication and of enhanced fetal surveillance. The judgment by the care provider was that neither was needed at that time and that continued follow-up would occur. The following devastating event supports the patient's concerns and raises directly the question why the care provider did not listen to the patient.

In this counseling session, the basic principles that follow provide a path for controlling the discussion while providing education. The initial part of the conversation allows the care provider to establish that the counseling session will continue as long as the family members have questions. It is appropriate then for the care provider to express sadness and condolences for the bad outcome. The care provider may initiate the conversation by indicating that some people in the midst of their anguish would feel great anger, and if that feeling is there, it is important that it be discussed and the underlying cause evaluated thoroughly. In this case, which involves the possibility that additional monitoring of both patient and baby could have changed the outcome, it is appropriate to address that issue specifically. Finally, the family should be provided the information that this type of case humbles the care provider, but that the knowledge generated from this event may alert future care providers to the possibility of such an outcome and possibly a change in obstetric management.

Basic Principles

- At the beginning of the counseling session, establish that you have set aside as much time for this meeting as the family feels is appropriate.

- Acknowledge your feelings of sadness, and offer condolences for the bad outcome.

- Use third-person counseling to define the focus of their anger.

- If your care produced that adverse outcome, admit it. If that association is questionable, state that as well.

- Portray the lessons learned as valuable for other patients in your practice and other care providers in your practice as well.

- Document the discussions.

Here is how the actual conversation might go:

Points to Cover	The Conversation
Protected time for discussion.	Mrs. L., I appreciate the fact that your family came in so that I could meet with all of you to discuss your baby's death. I have changed my schedule this afternoon to allow as much time as you and your family feel is necessary to discuss these issues. [It is appropriate to review for the family and the patient the sequence of events leading up to the death and labor and delivery.]
Express sadness, and search for anger.	There are many circumstances in obstetrics in which one might feel great sadness but also enormous anger that such an event occurred. If this is a feeling that you are having, then I would like to spend some time discussing that specifically. [At this point, a family member is more likely than the patient to attack the care provider verbally indicating outrage that such an event could occur under the presumed knowledge of a trained care provider. The care provider's response might go as follows:] I can understand and appreciate your anger.

Points to Cover	The Conversation
Be honest.	As I review the sequence of events, at the time that J.L. showed a slight rise in her blood pressure, it was not in the range that I felt needed treatment. The baby's growth had been appropriate, indicating that the intrauterine environment was supportive of a normal baby's development. Unfortunately, it now appears that J.L.'s blood pressure rapidly rose and that the abruption that we now think was linked to the baby's death probably did result from that elevated blood pressure. These are events that humble all of us and remind us that we do not control all biological events. In retrospect, I cannot say for certain that placing J.L. on an antihypertensive medication or even doing antepartum testing for fetal health could have warned us that the mother and baby were at risk. Nonetheless, I must confess that had we initiated both when her blood pressure was beginning to rise, we might have been provided warning that the baby was in trouble and perhaps we might have been able to act in a more aggressive manner.
Repeat the facts to family members.	[A pause may allow the family to reiterate their anger once again, or at least begin to acknowledge that the signs and symptoms preceding the final event may not have been as clear as they thought based on the information they were provided. Also, it may be valuable to repeat the sequence of events such that the family hears the same clinical course as was described at the beginning of the session. Finally, the conversation continues.]

Points to Cover	The Conversation
Describe programmatic changes.	This type of clinical situation continues to remind us that we have much to learn about the obstetric course of women who present with blood pressure elevations. It inspires research to learn why these events occur and what we can do in the future to avert them. My partners and I have discussed your case in depth and hope that the lessons learned will help improve patient care in similar cases in the future.
Restate the initial rationale for management.	I have given this a lot of thought. If I could do it again, I may have started the fetal monitoring earlier. I am not sure that we would have detected a problem soon enough because these tests are not perfect. It is not clear also whether such tests or even medication would have changed the outcome. Placental abruptions are linked to a number of conditions and health risks. Hypertension has a recognized association with placental abruption. Whether antihypertensive medication would have reduced that risk, however, is not clear. Nonetheless, I probably would have placed you on blood-pressure-lowering medication since your blood pressure was a little high. [Restating awareness of the patient's condition prior to the loss and the decision not to place her on antihypertensive medicine may be appropriate because it reestablishes the thought process that was in place initially].

Points to Cover	The Conversation
Offer to continue the conversation.	As we close this session, I understand that you will be continuing to talk to your other family members and perhaps your friends. New questions may come up. I would offer that if you would like a second counseling session, I would arrange my schedule. Then we can review the clinical course and the decisions that were made and the thought process behind those decisions. I will make my time available and will align it with any time that you think is appropriate. I thank all of you for coming in, and I repeat how sad I feel that such a terrible event has occurred.
Document.	[A thorough documentation of the discussion should be entered into the medical record.]

What do I say when a member of my group or department involved in a bad outcome refuses to meet with the patient or her family?

As chief of your obstetrics service, it is your custom to make ward rounds each morning. This morning, your usual routine is disrupted by the charge nurse, who describes to you a case that she feels is being handled poorly. She tells you that one of the four obstetricians in the department of your hospital last night had a bad case. His patient had been noncompliant throughout her pregnancy, the significance of which was made worse by her type II diabetes and her poor dietary compliance. This overweight woman arrived on the labor deck 5 centimeters dilated and then rapidly progressed to full dilation. The delivery was traumatic for both the woman and the physician, since a shoulder dystocia was encountered, requiring several minutes to effect the delivery. The 4700-gram baby boy now resides in the nursery with a fractured humerus and some seizure activity controlled with medication.

The charge nurse was informed this morning by the nurse who attended the delivery that the obstetrician was irate at the lack of responsibility that the patient took for this pregnancy. He commented in the hallway following the delivery that it was her irresponsibility that had placed him in the disturbing position of having to encounter the shoulder dystocia. The obstetrician also was overheard to say that the patient got what she deserved and that he had no interest in talking with her or her family about this event. Following the delivery, his anger was so intense that he was unable to converse with the family, and he left the hospital.

Armed with this information, you contact the obstetrician and arrange to have a meeting in your office that afternoon. Your purpose is to hear the obstetrician's side of the argument and, in your role as chief of obstetrics, to decrease the risks of a lawsuit as a result of poor communication with the family.

Just prior to the meeting you ask yourself:

- How should I introduce the issue?
- Can I get an unbiased description of the circumstances?
- How will I figure out why this care provider chose this approach with the family?
- How can we develop a course for resolving this impasse?
- What are my options for dealing with this individual?

This is a complex dilemma with tremendous opportunity for misinterpretation. Most group practices function as an extended family, crosscovering each other to provide time off from work, providing consultation, and generally serving as support for the many rigors created during the general practice of obstetrics. At first glance, an uninvolved member of the group may either admit relief behind the scenes that he or she was not involved in the case or express anger that this individual's decision not to meet with the patient and her family puts the entire group at litigious risk. Both attitudes create two challenges. Members who were relieved that they were not the responsible partner at the delivery may distance themselves from this case, an unfortunate stance that is likely to influence the group's future interactions down the road. Members angered by this posturing also may distance themselves from the involved individual out of a feeling of an inability to control how the involved member is resolving this issue; ultimately, this stance may translate into an increased lack of confidence in the clinical skills of the involved member. In this particular case, neither punitive actions nor distancing offers resolution for the other members of the group or direction to the involved individual.

Resolving this case demands that one individual from the group, perhaps the chairperson of the department or a senior member of the group, arrange to meet with the involved individual to open up a discourse on why he has chosen a path for addressing this patient's needs that seems incongruous with good medical teaching. The conversation should explore the issues, how the patient and family perceived the delivery, and their response during and after discharge. Armed with this information, the senior member, now playing a role of mediator and possibly conciliator, must query the reasons behind the physician's actions because they seem to conflict with that which is intuitive based on the circumstances. Is the department member afraid that he erred? Should more have been done to counsel the patient during the pregnancy? Is the physician fearful for his life? Or, in the worst scenario, is he arrogant regarding the outcome and believes he is above reproach? It is only this last scenario that may offer little remedy other than to reeducate the individual regarding his liability in this case and the importance of communicating to the patient and her family a proper description of the events.

Seeking input from the family as to their perception of the events becomes fundamental to the dialogue. The care provider must be dealt with through group dynamics in which the partners of the practice, through their interaction, either encourage a softening of this positioning or threaten separation from this individual because he has become a liability to the group. A compromise may be reached if the individual is willing to seek professional help in interpersonal communications and anger management through internal or external programs. Peer review for corrective actions also may assist him.

Basic Principles

- One individual, be it the department chairperson or a senior practice member, should take the lead as the negotiator-conciliator.
- Get all of the details of the case.
- Initiate the conversation with the individual by identifying the strengths of his clinical skills, but then indicate that the approach this individual has chosen with this family that has incurred a bad outcome is inconsistent with good medical care and opens up the opportunities for liability.
- Seek to understand the physician's impression of the family's reaction to the event and the potential sources for misconception or misinterpretation.
- Address directly with the involved clinician the reasons that he feels compelled not to meet with the family.
- In the conversation with the care provider, identify whether his actions result from personal fear, guilt, or arrogance.
- If needed, offer to negotiate between the family and the care provider.
- Address fear or guilt in a group session in which the patient and her family, with the senior faculty member as a negotiator or a moderator, discuss the issues of the case and the family's interpretation.
- Direct the physician to choose options for communicating with the family.
- Document the discussion.

The actual conversation might go as follows:

Points to Cover	The Conversation
Take the lead as the negotiator.	Dr. G., I have asked you in my capacity as chief of service [or chairperson of the department] to discuss with me the tough case that you had to manage last night that resulted in a shoulder dystocia and a depressed newborn.

Points to Cover	The Conversation
Identify strengths.	I am sure this event was very traumatic for you, as it was for the family. I have always thought of you as a good clinician, but your approach to the family seems inconsistent with good medical care.
Provide a plausible explanation for behavior.	Dr. G., I can understand where this type of experience can humble even a senior physician. Perhaps your reticence to meet with the family stems from your feelings of vulnerability made worse by your patient's noncompliant behavior. [At this point, Dr. G. may express those feelings, thereby allowing him to suggest that it is time to sit with the family.] I can imagine these intense feelings of anger that you are expressing could result from your concerns that you did not pursue this patient's behavior more aggressively in order to make her a more responsible patient. Is this true? [This too may generate a line of conversation leading to the recognition that meeting with the patient is by far the best way to reduce the risks of a malpractice suit.]
Offer to be a negotiator.	Dr. G., sometimes it becomes necessary when such an impasse occurs for someone like myself to sit in such a session and to offer a moderate voice, but also to serve as moderator in the discussions. I would be willing to do that if you would like. I believe in my capacity as protector of this institution that some form of communication with the family and the patient needs to be initiated. I would understand if you decided yourself to take this initiative. If not, I believe I need to work with you to find some way in which you can be

Points to Cover	The Conversation
Offer to be a negotiator. (cont.)	comfortable with the conversation. The patient and her family must be given the opportunity to discuss their side of the issues. Their questions may be easily answered, and the conversation may resolve misunderstandings that otherwise will be left intact and may lead to a subsequent lawsuit.
Encouragement and advice.	[The conversation may wind down, but some type of encouraging statement should be made to the individual physician.] Dr. G., I would like you to think about the options I have laid out. I will respect your decision either to meet with the family alone or to involve me in some capacity. They too have incurred a traumatic event, and I believe the very best way to serve them is not to withdraw but to be upfront as care providers. I would like to follow up with you tomorrow to hear how you view this and which course of action you would like to take. Again, thank you for coming into my office and talking about this very complex situation.
Document	[A thorough documentation of the discussion should be entered into the medical record.]

What do I say in response to a patient's inquiry when she interprets the use of slang by care providers as minimizing the significance of a bad outcome?

T.J. is a thirty-year-old G2, P1 whose uneventful pregnancy culminates at term with spontaneous onset of labor and an uneventful delivery. The newborn exhibits seizure activity immediately after delivery and is taken to the neonatal intensive care nursery for evaluation. Family members, obviously distraught, are comforted by your comments that the pediatricians taking care of their baby are well versed in evaluating these types of symptoms and surely will provide important information as soon as it is available.

Later that day, a family member takes the elevator to the cafeteria for a cup of coffee. In the elevator also are two young pediatric residents from the neonatal intensive care nursery. The family member overhears one resident say to the other, "Did you see the new admission to our nursery? I think it's a FLK." The other resident indicates that she is not familiar with that abbreviation. "What does that mean?" she says. The first resident, in a somewhat jocular matter, answers, "It means a funny looking kid."

The family member, standing in the back of the elevator, is outraged by the insensitivity of the statement and immediately calls your office and requests that the family speak with you immediately. Later that afternoon, you meet the family and are presented the elevator scenario. As you listen to their story, you ask yourself:

- How do I respond to the family's outrage?
- How do I explain why these young caregivers appeared so insensitive?
- Why would they use slang as a defense?
- How do I get the conversation back on track?
- What sort of education should I suggest these care providers be provided?

In this scenario, the human element of medicine has been exposed. The use of slang by young professionals, either students or young faculty, offers protection against the emotional fear that failure or death imposes on young care providers. Young people enter medicine with an idealized version of what medicine is all about. Few have experienced the personal despair or tragedy that would prepare them to be comfortable in the presence of a patient who has encountered such tragedy. Slang offers a protective wall; by using the dark side of humor, young care providers avoid the emotional risk of becoming involved and therefore personally traumatized along with the patient to whom they are providing care.

Your discussion with this family must be straightforward and honest. A full apology for the insensitive statements made offers the initial lead into a more fundamental discussion about the care of their baby. Most patients, if counseled appropriately, can understand how young professionals in medicine could make insensitive statements without realizing their impact. By acknowledging this weakness in the education and maturity of young care providers, the discussion then can shift to the baby and away from a continued discussion about the insensitive comments or the insensitivity of the young care providers. The final comments in the counseling session should include your appreciation that the family members can understand this dilemma and that it will not happen again. It should also be stated that these young care providers will be told about the impact of their insensitive comments.

Basic Principles

- Apologize for the insensitive statements that were made.
- Reaffirm the fact that the baby's care is being carried out by professionals who know what they are doing.
- Explain how younger professionals in medicine frequently use slang to distance themselves emotionally from the harsh realities of medicine.
- Repeat your apology for the insensitive statements.
- Describe how these young care providers will be counseled so that they will not repeat this offense.
- Document the discussion.

Here is how the conversation might go:

Points to Cover	The Conversation
Express appreciation.	T.J., I thank you and your family for finding time to meet with me so that we can address concerns that you have regarding the comments that were said in the elevator about your baby, John, by two young care providers. I personally have discussed John's condition with my colleagues in the neonatal intensive care nursery and they assure me that as soon as all of the tests are completed, they will meet with you, and if you would like, with me, to discuss your son's condition.

Points to Cover	The Conversation
Apologize.	Thank you for bringing this incident to my attention. I apologize to you for the insensitive comments that these care providers made.
Explain the quality assurance issue.	The comments should not have been made, and the individuals who were involved have been properly counseled so that they will not do it again.
Describe how slang protects young care providers.	It is my observation that the use of slang in medicine often provides protection to young care providers against the emotional toll of confronting illness and death regularly. Few of these individuals have experienced personal loss or grief, and it is understandable that they would not be prepared to respond to the grief of others. Slang distances these young care providers from the emotional trauma that caring for a sick patient can create. As they become more experienced with illness and death, they will abandon these types of defenses.
Note the idealism of young care providers.	Young people enter medicine with a very idealized version of the medical profession, and they are unprepared for their first encounters with serious illness and the grieving response associated with it. These young professionals seldom have experienced sufficient life crises themselves to be armed properly to respond to these events when they happen to patients for whom they are caring.
Reaffirm your apology.	I do not offer this explanation to you in any way as an effort to defend the actions of these individuals. I only ask you to consider my interpretation as to why young professionals would make such insensitive comments. If there are other issues that

Points to Cover	The Conversation
Reaffirm your apology. (cont.)	develop while your son is in the hospital, I hope you will feel comfortable to contact me so that we can arrange time to talk.
Document.	[A thorough documentation of the discussion should be entered into the medical record.]

What do I say when under the influence of fatigue, I am short-tempered with a family member and then something bad happens?

J.D., a patient of yours, is a twenty-three-year-old G1, P1, who now is two days postpartum from a cesarean section for failure to progress in labor. J.D.'s medical history is complicated by morbid obesity, type II diabetes mellitus, mild chronic hypertension, and frequent urinary tract infections. Her pregnancy progressed unremarkably until thirty-eight weeks' gestation, when she went into labor. The labor became dysfunctional when she was 6 centimeters dilated, and despite Pitocin augmentation, she made no further progress. A cesarean section was carried out, productive of a healthy 4380-gram male named James.

Through the night proceeding this second postoperative day, you have been very busy. You began the night with three patients in labor. One delivered at 1:00 A.M., one patient at 3:30 A.M., and another patient at 5:30 A.M. Despite your effort to clear your morning office schedule, several patients need to be seen, and you agree reluctantly to see them in the office that morning.

Before going to the office, you round on J.D., who appears to be recovering nicely from her surgery. Her blood pressure is elevated but does not seem to you to require antihypertensive medications. Although she is groggy in this early morning visit, she appears to be stable.

While at the office, you are called at 9:30 A.M. by a family member who expresses concern that J.D. remains quite sluggish. Despite feeling fatigued, you respond politely and courteously that you just made rounds and are quite sure that J.D. is doing well and most likely is just sleepy from tossing and turning through the night. At 11:45 A.M., you go to the hospital and make brief rounds on J.D., also noting that she is somewhat difficult to arouse. Her vital signs, however, remain stable. The family approaches you, again expressing their concerns, and this time you are somewhat agitated, but you still remain calm in your answers that J.D. is doing fine.

You then go home to catch a few hours of sleep, only to be awakened by a family member who is calling with grave concerns about J.D.'s condition. At this point, your courteousness is overcome by your fatigue. You snap at the family member on the telephone that you just saw J.D. today, that she is doing fine, and that the family should calm down and stop worrying. You even go so far as to say that people who are not in medicine should not be making medical judgments and that you know what is best for J.D. and wish to get a little sleep, because you are very tired.

At 5:00 P.M., you are awakened by a nurse on the floor who informs you that J.D. has just arrested and that resuscitation is ongoing but has not produced any positive results. You dress rapidly and rush to the hospital. When you arrive, the head nurse tells you that resuscitation was discontinued. J.D. has been declared dead. The family members are so angry that they refuse to meet with you. When they are approached as to whether they will seek an autopsy, they reject this offer, and the comments you hear from them as they rapidly walk down the hall are that they will get even.

The next day, you call the family members and state clearly the need for you to meet with them. To your surprise and despite their intense anger at you, they agree reluctantly to such a meeting. When they arrive in your office, they place an eight- by ten-inch photograph of their daughter in front of you, thus setting the initial tone of the discussions.

You ask yourself:

- How do I begin the conversation?
- How do I control the level of anger?

- How do I apologize for my snap responses and yet defend my clinical judgment without being confrontational?
- How do I engage them in a retrospective review of the care? What would they have wanted done?
- Can I make anything positive out of this negative event?

This is a scenario that care providers who work long hours dread most. Medicine is not a science but an art form, and in medicine, events can occur that may in fact not be preventable. The impact of such an event is made that much greater when the care provider's interactions with family members are compromised by fatigue or the perceived notion that the care provider has no time to be attentive to family members' concerns. When fatigue overcomes good judgment and drives one to lash out at a family member, the scene is set for calamity. For family members unaccustomed to medicine, it is difficult for them to understand that the care provider has other responsibilities. They also may not be able to judge the impact of long hours on anyone's ability to be courteous. Nonetheless, there is never an excuse for a care provider to respond in a rude or thoughtless way.

The meeting, which draws on all of the interpersonal skills that the care provider can generate, begins with a review of the events of the case in order to establish the facts. This is the opportunity to acknowledge that the fatigue had a strong influence on the care provider's responses to the family's request. This statement alone may elicit anger from the family. If so, ample time should be allowed for this type of discourse. The care provider, however, should repeat the sequence of events if in fact management was appropriate but an unexpected event occurred. This statement most likely will regenerate anger as the family clearly reminds you that they were aware that something was happening, even though all of the vital signs were demonstrating something else. They may even express frustration that no additional tests were done in the hour or so before their daughter's death. In your discussion, you ultimately may seek from them how they would have preferred you to respond. This engages the family in the discussion and may clarify the issues that lie beneath their anger. If the family indicates that additional testing should have been done, you may be able to respond that the standard tests done for a postoperative patient were indicating that the patient was stable. If the family wants an accounting of your activities during that period, this line of inquiry may allow you to provide them information about your other responsibilities or your need for sleep after a long night at the hospital.

If the family asks what is going to happen now, this may be an opportunity to use the death of their loved one as a basic principle by which other doctors in your practice can become more aware of the art of communication through the eyes of the patient's family. You may suggest that this event will be used in a grand rounds to teach the principles of communicating with the family.

The family still may harbor such anger as to threaten you with a lawsuit. If you believe that nothing could have been done differently, you may wish to advise them that lawsuits frequently are extended over years, thereby drawing out their sadness for an extended period of time that will not undo the events that have occurred. While this may not lead to their agreeing with you, it may give them pause to consider later whether this type of action is really indicated. Educating them regarding the health issues of their daughter may provide them information that initially they did not have.

At the end of the discussion, you should thank them for coming to your office under stress to discuss such a difficult issue. It is appropriate to express your condolences for their daughter's death and the fact that you are more aware than ever before how important it is to listen to a family's concerns, since often families know more about their individual loved ones than do the care providers.

Basic Principles
- Review the facts with the family.
- Express condolences.
- Acknowledge that fatigue may have compromised the communication with the family.
- Clarify the importance of family input.

- Comment on how lessons learned from this event and the role of fatigue in a clinical judgment may be brought to the attention of department members through a quality assurance session or a grand rounds.
- Document the conversation, the individuals at the meeting, the issues that were covered, the mood of the conversation, and any future steps involving the family to address questions that remained unanswered.

Here is how this conversation might go. Note that it uses each of the components of the "Feared Factor" and the elements of full disclosure to address the anger that is evident in the family's comments:

Points to Cover	The Conversation
Review the facts.	I appreciate the time that you have taken to meet with me and to discuss the death of J.D. We have reviewed the sequence of events leading up to her death, and I can summarize that as follows. [The details of the care provided during the hours prior to the death are described in detail and compassionately.]
Explain the process of care.	In reviewing the care that your daughter received, we relied heavily on the laboratory tests and vital signs that were obtained in the hours prior to her death. Those measures, in retrospect, gave us false reassurance that her condition was stable and that the risks for a catastrophic event were minimal.
Acknowledge the family's concerns.	That said, I realize that you expressed concern regarding your daughter's condition several times in the hours preceding her death. I also realize that while initially I considered those comments to reflect your lack of medical knowledge, in retrospect I understand now how concerned you were and that your concerns ultimately proved to be correct.

Points to Cover	The Conversation
Explain how the facts were acquired.	In anticipation of this meeting, we brought all the care providers together to review your daughter's care and to determine if there were any signs that we missed that might have helped us provide alternative management. Unfortunately, we do not find that type of evidence.
Apologize for your short temper.	That, however, does not excuse my short-tempered comments to you as you were expressing your concerns about your daughter's condition. During the night preceding your daughter's death, I was involved in the care of a number of obstetric patients. My reaction to your concerns, in retrospect, was influenced by my own fatigue. While I do not feel that my short-tempered comments affected the care that your daughter received, the tone of my comments clearly was unprofessional, and for that I apologize.
Engage the family.	Even as I have examined carefully the events leading up to your daughter's death, I would ask you if there were requests that you made or medical tests that you believe should have been carried out that would have provided us insight into the severity of her condition. [This question brings the family into the discussion of the management and provides insight as to the specific concerns that they had and that they felt were not addressed.]
Discuss the issue of fatigue in medicine.	As you know, the long hours that medical care providers spend have both a positive and a negative side. The obvious positive side is the ability to provide more care to more patients. The downside is the effect that fatigue has on our ability to sustain activity. You have asked me if fatigue played a role in your daughter's care. I believe it did not.

Points to Cover	The Conversation
Describe programmatic changes.	Our department nonetheless has discussed the issue of fatigue and its role in medical judgment, and we are considering reducing the number of hours that a staff physician can practice before he or she is required to seek some level of rest or sleep. I regret that your daughter's death has generated this type of discussion and the need for us to review our policy of sustained care. Nonetheless, medicine advances on one front through technological invention and another front through programmatic change in response to adverse outcomes and discussions such as this one that we are having today.
Thank the family.	I very much appreciate the effort that you have made to spend time with me, and again I offer my condolences on your daughter's death. Her death will change the way we practice medicine in this department, and in some sad way, I thank you for that.
Document.	[A thorough documentation of the discussion should be entered into the medical record.]

CHAPTER 5

Conversations to Educate

What should I say when someone has written an entry into the record that is inconsistent with the information conveyed to the patient and family?

J.L. is a twenty-five-year-old G2, P1 who presents at term in active labor. Because she is a gestational diabetic, her baby is known to be on the large side, but not so large as to require a primary cesarean section. After the patient has been in the second stage of labor for three hours, the fetal heart rate begins to demonstrate deep decelerations consistent with repeated umbilical cord compression. The attending physician and the third-year resident perform a series of forceps maneuvers. When it becomes apparent that J.L. is incapable of delivering vaginally, a stat cesarean section is carried out, productive of a depressed newborn girl with Apgar scores of 1, 1, 3, and 8 at one, five, ten, and fifteen minutes, respectively. In the neonatal intensive care nursery, the baby demonstrates seizure activity and ultimately is discharged on phenobarbital, but with concerns regarding the impact of intrauterine hypoxemia on long-term development. The physician responsible for the delivery is so distraught that he admits to you, his partner, that he is incapable of sitting with the family. Despite your encouragement to the contrary, he asks if you will perform this task.

You review the medical record in an effort to understand the sequence of events better, and you find that the first-year resident has dictated the discharge summary as "outlet forceps were applied, however, patient was unable to deliver infant with low forceps." The operative note, handwritten by a second-year resident peripheral to the case, was "cesarean section for failure to descend." The third-year resident, who actually was involved in the forceps application, did not write a note, and the staff physician wrote, "Left oxiput transverse, trial of labor attempted, but failed as the fetal head was at minus one station." The nursing notes indicate, "17:25 hours forceps applied, 17:29 forceps reapplied, 17:35 doctor discussing cesarean section with patient."

You are about to meet with the family to provide an interpretation of the maneuvers that led to the baby's delivery, and you recognize that the entries in the medical record are inconsistent, thereby greatly compromising the conversation that is about to take place. Your challenge is to get an accurate picture of what transpired and respond appropriately to a request by your colleague to carry out the conversation that he or she is unable to at this time.

You ask yourself:

- How can I be sure that my facts are correct?
- What general approach should I choose with the family?
- How do I explain the absence of their care provider?
- How can I explain the discrepancies in the medical record?

The basic principles of this challenge are to get the facts correct before having the conversation with the family. Because of the discrepancies you noted in the medical record, your first step should be an immediate request for a fact-finding conference of all participating care providers. This should be a closed session, partially to offer the opportunity for the care providers to express their emotional reaction to the outcome but also to get the facts correct from each person. It is understandable that in a teaching environment where multiple care providers are involved, one individual may document in the chart while another may have actually participated in the care. In this closed conference with the attending physician and the involved residents and nurses, the details must be carefully collected as a formal quality assurance process. This exchange provides protection for the information without making judgment about the care. This information should be part of the quality assurance process improvement or peer review file, begun as a routine in any adverse outcome by the hospital risk management.

Once the information has been collected, a time should be established to sit down with the family members in order to detail the events of the case and explain the adverse outcome.

Each of the steps described for the "Feared Factor" (see page 57) should be used. A review of the facts, what was done to assemble them correctly, and why the physician who provided the services is unable to be at this conversation need to be spelled out. Expressing sympathy for the outcome, searching for sources of anger, requiring the patient to recite back her understanding of the events, searching for other issues among extended family, and finally documenting the case are a part of the subsequent conversation.

It should be acknowledged to the family that there are inconsistent entries in the medical record by different people involved to a greater or lesser degree in J.L.'s management. This open disclosure reduces the chances that later on, these differences in data entry will be used in a confrontational way if the family seeks legal action. Thank the family for their understanding of the complex manner in which a hospital record is constructed, and document the conversation.

Basic Principles

- Convene a fact-finding meeting with all of the care providers before the counseling session with the family.
- Arrange for a conference with the family.
- Explain why the attending physician is not at the counseling session.
- Use the "Feared Factor" approach for counseling the family.
- Acknowledge that the entries in the chart offer different interpretations of the events.
- Explain the different levels of care providers involved in entering information in the medical record.

- Thank J.L. and her family for allowing you to explain the complexities of how a medical record is constructed.
- Document the discussion.

Here is how the conversation might go:

Points to Cover	The Conversation
Get the facts.	[Prior to the meeting with the family, bring all of the care providers into a closed session in which the facts of the delivery are discussed and discrepancies in the record are reviewed. In this session, you may be surprised at the emotional impact of this event on the various care providers. The attending nurse may express with some anger her reactions when several efforts at applying forceps were carried out instead of moving toward performing a cesarean section. The involved residents also may express their concerns and even fear that involvement in a case in which they did not have complete control could place them in professional jeopardy. This emotional disclosure offers some release from the tensions created among the various care providers involved in a bad outcome, and it may help to explain the discrepancies in the record. A meeting is then set with J.L. and her family to discuss the events of the delivery.]
Bring the family together.	J.L., I thank you and your family for coming to my office to discuss your baby daughter's delivery. Dr. F., who was the attending physician for your delivery, is not here today. He has asked me to coordinate this meeting, because he is too saddened and upset over the outcome to be comfortable to be here. Perhaps at a later time if you would like to meet with him personally, we could accommodate that.

What Do I Say?

Points to Cover	The Conversation
Use the "Feared Factor."	[The conversation follows the pattern of the "Feared Factor" to discuss the events of the delivery and your concerns regarding the outcome for the baby. The final component of the discussion focuses on the discrepancies in the medical record.]
Admit the contradictions in charting.	J.L., in reviewing the chart in preparation for our discussion, I came across a number of entries, some of which were not exactly in agreement. I have met with each of the care providers in order to get the facts correct, and those are the facts that we have just discussed. What often is not appreciated is that notations in a medical record are entered by a number of individuals, some of whom are directly involved in the patient's care and some of whom are asked to place additional data in the record for the sake of completeness. It is my interpretation that differences in notes entered into the record reflected the opinions of different individuals, some of whom were more peripherally involved in the delivery of your daughter.
Restate the purpose of the meeting.	I hope that this counseling session has been helpful for you, because I am aware of how difficult it has been for you to discuss your daughter's condition. Nonetheless, I felt that we should sit and review the record to make sure that all of our facts were correct.
Document.	[The medical record should include an entry about the conversation.]

In this case, a second session with J.L.'s obstetrician and J.L.'s family was arranged. The issue of charting did not surface. The conversation centered on the maneuvers used to attempt a vaginal delivery and the decision to proceed to a cesarean section. The family mood was considerate and appreciative of the extra time and effort taken to meet with them.

What do I say when a patient who has had a bad outcome tells me that she wants to bring her lawyer to our counseling session?

You are making inpatient rounds and enter the room of D.J. She is a twenty-nine-year-old G1, P1 whose prenatal course was complicated by preterm labor at twenty-six weeks' gestation that did not respond to tocolytic medication. In late labor, D.J.'s fetus suddenly exhibited an abrupt bradycardia to sixty beats per minute, and a stat cesarean section was carried out. Personnel from pediatrics were in attendance and provided appropriate resuscitation, but D.J.'s baby, now in the neonatal intensive care nursery, exhibits some seizure activity.

D.J. is understandably upset as you approach her in her hospital room on the day of discharge. It is your policy to bring such patients back into your office in the first week after discharge to review the events of the hospitalization and to answer questions that your patient or her family may have. You offer this to D.J. She responds, "I want to bring a lawyer to that session." Momentarily, you are caught off-guard. No patient in the past has made this type of veiled threat. As you quickly gather your thoughts, you ask yourself:

- Is this appropriate?
- Is D.J. overstepping her bounds?
- What are my rights as a physician who is offering such a counseling session?
- Is there a counteroffer that I can submit to D.J. if the concept of having a lawyer present appears to me as intrusive and possibly obstructive to good communication?

This seemingly innocent request by a patient who is about to be counseled for a bad event introduces limitations to good communication. The patient may believe that having her lawyer at the counseling session will ensure that the discussion will be accurate and balanced. The care provider in this case may acknowledge initially that it is the patient's right to have a lawyer in any setting in which the patient is receiving information. The key to this conversation, however, is to educate the patient that the presence of the lawyer stifles any free-flowing communication and mandates that both sides of this communication have legal representation. When provided with the information that the presence of a lawyer essentially will block the process of communicating accurate facts and sharing emotional responses, most patients will agree not to require legal counsel at this conversation.

Basic Principles

- Clarify that the presence of a lawyer on the patient's side mandates that a lawyer represent the care provider and that you put your insurer on notice.
- Notify the risk manager about the conversation. If the patient agrees not to bring a lawyer, this too should be part of the information conveyed to the risk manager.
- The presence of lawyers for both parties will block the opportunity to communicate factual information and, more important, to seek emotional responses to the catastrophic event.
- Armed with the knowledge that the presence of lawyers most likely will eliminate any ability to communicate freely, the patient in most cases will elect not to have legal representation at the first meeting.
- Document carefully the conversation leading to the decision not to have legal representation.

Here is how the conversation might go:

Points to Cover	The Conversation
Clarify the role of a lawyer.	Mrs. D.J., I understand that you have requested that your lawyer be present at our counseling session. It is always your right to have legal representation. However, if you require a lawyer at that session, then I will need to have a lawyer represent me, since we need a balanced atmosphere for communicating.

Points to Cover	The Conversation
Explain the obstacles to communicating.	Your lawyer may not allow you to ask questions freely, because those questions may disclose misunderstanding or other issues that will work against you. My lawyer may not allow me to answer your questions freely, a right that you have as my patient. And because of the presence of the two lawyers, you and I will not be able to communicate openly and share our feelings about this terrible event.
Focus on the facts.	[The patient considers the issues presented. D.J. then says:] I have listened to your argument and I agree that it is more important for me to seek information regarding this event than for me to be concerned about legal representation at this time. If I still feel that I need legal representation after our first meeting, then I will request it. [The care provider then may respond as follows:] If after our discussion you feel that way, then that is your privilege. Nonetheless, I would like to make sure that you have the facts before you make such a decision.
Document.	[A thorough documentation of the discussion should be entered into the medical record.]

What do I say when a patient, after good advice from me to the contrary, has mandated a clinical course that results in an adverse consequence?

S.M. is a G2, P1 whose first pregnancy resulted in a cesarean section for a 4300-gram fetus. In your prenatal counseling, you offer her the options of a repeat cesarean section or a vaginal birth after cesarean section (VBAC) and explain the advantages and disadvantages of each. You indicate that the advantages of a cesarean section are that it can be carried out in a timely manner. The negative is a longer rehabilitation postoperatively and a small chance of infection or bleeding as a result of the surgery. Another advantage of the VBAC is that recovery is more rapid following delivery. You also explain to the patient that with a VBAC, there is a small risk of uterine rupture and if that does occur, it could place the baby at risk for injury or death.

S.M. labors all day and makes poor but steady progress. You approach her several times during the labor suggesting that a cesarean section might be needed, but she rejects that idea. The fetal heart rate has been documented to be stable throughout the labor process. At 8 centimeters, however, there is a sudden fetal bradycardia. A stat cesarean section is carried out under general anesthesia, but a uterine rupture is encountered, with the male fetus extruding into the abdominal cavity. Despite aggressive resuscitation, the newborn fails to respond. At twenty minutes, resuscitation is discontinued, and the baby is declared dead.

A few hours after the surgery, once S.M. has recovered fully from the anesthesia, you sit down next to her bedside. You think:

- How can I begin the conversation?
- How can I be sympathetic and yet reiterate how her decision and my advice to her differed?
- Can we find a middle road to discuss this outcome?
- How can I diffuse my patient's guilt feelings?

This is a conversation that requires finesse and yet must end with a win-win situation. The most feared consequence of a VBAC now has been realized and most likely resulted from the poor labor progress. S.M.'s decision to press on with the labor was against your advice. One can only imagine the guilt that this type of situation engenders.

The basic objectives of this conversation are to acknowledge the event, express respect for the patient's ability to choose her own health destination, and yet balance this with the fact that this was not the clinical course that you recommended. The care provider in this case can acknowledge that this was not the clinical course he or she would have supported and perhaps should have been more insistent that this clinical path not be taken. This maneuver maintains the patient's control (VBAC is an accepted management) while also restating the objectives of the care provider's advice (poor labor progress should have prompted an earlier cesarean section).

Basic Principles

- Express sadness over the clinical event and describe briefly the sequence.

- Establish that by today's medical standards, patients are being given more control over their health decisions. Although this is a positive step, it can produce adverse medical consequences.

- Restate that many women choose to have a VBAC after considering the advantages and disadvantages of a cesarean section versus a VBAC.

- Connect this thought with the fact that it is impossible to identify who really is at risk for uterine rupture with a VBAC.

- Acknowledge that these types of dilemmas may create guilt, but that it reminds both the care provider and the patient that we do not control all events in health.

- Document the discussion.

This conversation could be conducted within hours after the cesarean section or as soon as the family is able to be present in the patient's postpartum room. Here is how the actual conversation might go:

Points to Cover	The Conversation
Express condolences and educate.	Mrs. S.M., I am deeply saddened by the sequence of events that occurred and led to your baby's death. [This statement alone may bring overwhelming grief that requires a period of minutes or longer before the conversation can continue.] As you know, you were progressing slowly in labor, and we had the opportunity to talk on several occasions about whether we should proceed with a cesarean

Points to Cover	The Conversation
Express condolences and educate. (cont.)	section. When the baby's heart rate suddenly dropped, we rushed you to the operating room, which I know must have been a frightening experience for you, and performed a cesarean section under general anesthesia. Your uterus had ruptured from the labor, and your baby son was out in the abdomen. Because your son had been expelled from the uterus, he was deprived of oxygen, and that is why the resuscitation was unsuccessful. I am so saddened by this event. [Here again, a period of time may need to lapse where the patient grieves.]
Explain autonomy.	Medical care today has changed a lot from what it was thirty years ago. Back then, it might have been appropriate for me to tell you, the patient, what type of care you would receive. Today, medical care is a negotiation that respects your wishes and tries to fit them within the confines of good medical care.
Express support for standards and awareness of risks.	It is understandable when one hears the advantages and disadvantages of a cesarean section versus a VBAC that one would choose the VBAC. Sadly, we do not have any test that can help us to define which patient is at risk for uterine rupture and the possibility that her baby might die. We include this in our consent to indicate the seriousness by which we take this process. Still, at least at present, we support the ability of a woman to choose VBAC over repeat cesarean section. It is quite understandable that one may reflect back on this and feel guilt at the decisions that one made. That step, however, may be taking more responsibility on yourself than is justified. When you chose to have a

Points to Cover	The Conversation
Express support for standards and awareness of risks. (cont.)	VBAC, you and I entered into an agreement indicating that while we both understood the risks, we both understood the acceptability of this type of labor process.
Express humility.	The fact that you experienced the most dreaded consequence of a VBAC, while very sad, reminds us that neither you nor I understand all events in medicine. We make our choices based on the best information at hand, and in the vast majority of cases, we experience good outcomes. I am deeply saddened that we did not experience that type of outcome this time.
Document.	[A thorough documentation of the discussion should be entered into the medical record.]

How honest should I be when a mistake is made in care but there is no adverse consequence?

You have just written orders to augment the labor of your patient, R.S., who is a twenty-four-year-old G1, P0 at thirty-nine weeks' gestation. The nurse preparing the Pitocin inadvertently places two ampules of Pitocin into 1000 cc of Ringer's lactate, thereby doubling the concentration of Pitocin that has been ordered. After the Pitocin has been infusing for thirty minutes, uterine activity rapidly increases and is brought to your attention. The Pitocin immediately is discontinued, and in the discussion with the nurse, the issue of the two ampules of Pitocin is identified. You now know that the nurse has been infusing Pitocin at twice the concentration that you ordered. Fortunately, the fetal heart rate was not affected by this overmedication. Nonetheless, you ask yourself:

- How honest should I be with the patient?
- Why should I say anything since no harm was done?
- How can I reassure my patient this will not happen again?
- Should I write down anything in the medical records?

122

There is only one way to manage this scenario, which challenges the basic integrity of our health care delivery system. Honesty is the foundation of health care. The patient should be informed of the error and, more important, provided information as to how, as a quality assurance issue, steps will be taken to help avoid this from occurring in the future.

The fact that there were no adverse consequences of the mishap is fortunate. By providing the patient full disclosure, the care provider maintains the very essence of honesty as an ongoing philosophy and draws the patient into the process of correcting this issue for future patients. This gesture of complete honesty, even as the issue of human error casts doubt momentarily on the quality of medicine provided, protects the trust that the patient seeks to place in her care provider.

In this scenario, a straightforward discussion of the error was provided to the patient. The consequences were spelled out clearly. Importantly, the ramifications of this discovery were stated in their most positive sense: a thorough departmentwide review of the protocol for Pitocin induction and the statement that because of the discovery of this error, future patients will not incur the same problems. Whenever a mistake is made and the mistake is brought to the attention of a patient, providing information that allows this person to understand that he or she may have helped someone in the future may offset the initial reaction of surprise and even lack of confidence in the care being provided.

Basic Principles

- State the event clearly to the patient.

- Acknowledge that no adverse consequences occurred.

- State the significance of the discovery, and indicate that the event would be used to review guidelines for care to prevent such an event from occurring in the future.

- Repeat the fact that the discovered event had no adverse consequences, but that the discovery will help in improving the overall care for patients.

- Document the discussion.

Here is how the conversation might go:

Points to Cover	The Conversation
State the event.	R.S., I have just completed a discussion with your nurse, who informs me that when the concentration of Pitocin was made to stimulate your labor, twice as much Pitocin was placed in the liquid bag as should have been. You may recall that shortly after we began the Pitocin, your uterine activity quickly increased, and we felt it necessary to stop the Pitocin. We examined the reasons for this, and that is when we discovered the problem.
Express lack of consequences.	Fortunately, we were monitoring your baby's heart rate and detected no evidence that your baby was placed under any stress because of the increased contractions. Nonetheless, this is a source of concern to us, and we felt compelled to bring it to your attention.
Describe the quality assurance component.	As a result, we now feel it is necessary to reevaluate our protocol for mixing Pitocin. Fortunately, there appears to be no adverse consequence from this mistake. Nonetheless, we will use this information to examine our protocol for Pitocin, and this may help some patient in the future.
Document.	[A thorough documentation of the discussion should be entered into the medical record.]

What do I say to a patient whose anger is based on a misperception of events?

R.B., a twenty-eight-year-old G2, P1 type 1 diabetic, has been poorly compliant with her diet and insulin regime throughout the pregnancy. Serial ultrasounds have demonstrated progressive fetal macrosomia. Following a third-trimester amniocentesis to confirm fetal lung maturity, R.B. is induced into labor. Labor proceeds uneventfully, but at delivery, a severe shoulder dystocia is encountered. The patient recounts later that there was a flurry of activity among the care providers in the delivery room, and a great deal of pulling. Following delivery, a full resuscitation was performed. The baby did not die but incurred prolonged hypoxemia that produced seizures in the neonatal intensive care nursery and a prolonged hospitalization.

The physician who delivered the baby later reported that her schedule made it difficult for her to get to the hospital to see the patient during the hospitalization. The physician recounts that even on the day of delivery, R.B.'s husband exhibited significant anger, which the physician felt would be directed at her or that could result in bodily injury. A week passes, and there is virtually no contact between the physician and the patient. The physician approaches you, describes the situation, and asks for your help.

You ask yourself:

- How can this impasse be broken?
- What type of counseling session should be scheduled, and who should be present?
- What series of questions should be asked to determine the focus of the husband's anger?
- What type of introductory statements should be used to introduce the conversation?
- How should the physician respond if the patient and her husband direct their anger toward the physician and even accuse the physician of mismanaging the delivery?
- What type of documentation should be placed in the chart at the time of delivery and then at the time of the postpartum counseling session?

The delivering obstetrician must be encouraged to call to schedule a meeting with the family immediately. If she so requests, you may serve as mediator to control the discussion and offer professional protection against bodily harm. In this conversation with the family, the six components of the "Feared Factor" apply (see chapter three).

The expression of condolence is an appropriate initial statement, followed by education as the principal component of this conversation. This unintended outcome, in which emergency measures were taken and in which inadequate time was available to counsel the family appropriately, easily leads to misunderstanding. For nonmedical people, attempting to understand emergency medical measures understandably is difficult. Acknowledging this difficulty is a central part of this conversation.

This case is complicated by the fact that this type 1 diabetic was poorly compliant with her diet and insulin regime. Exploring anger as a fundamental response by the family to the outcome is critical in this discussion. To do so, however, requires a strategy. Initially, the family has directed its anger at you. The anger from the husband's standpoint actually may be directed at his wife, who failed to take care of herself during the pregnancy and therefore was responsible in part for the fetal macrosomia that led to the shoulder dystocia. Searching for that source of anger may be challenging, since the husband consciously or unconsciously may not be comfortable to be that honest in the discussion. It is appropriate in such a conversation to use a third-person approach—for example: "Sometimes an outcome may be related to events during the pregnancy in which the woman could have made a difference by taking better care of herself. Is this an issue that you two have discussed?"

Basic Principles

- Use the "Feared Factor."

- Emphasize the value of educating the family.

- Explore the anger in search of its focus.

- Explain how emergencies in medicine often do not allow time for appropriate counseling.

- Explain how difficult it must be for nonmedical people to understand emergency-type medicine.

- Thank the family for meeting with you.

- Document the discussion.

After the initial discussion with you, the obstetrician decides to meet with the family without you, but appreciates your advice.

Points to Cover	The Conversation
Provide the facts.	R.B., thank you for finding time to allow us to sit down to discuss the difficult delivery that you experienced. The events that transpired are as follows. [A detailed discussion of the delivery should be given to set the facts straight.] R.B., I have talked with the physicians in the neonatal intensive care nursery, and they have provided me information about your baby's condition. [A short discussion of your understanding of the baby's condition is appropriate.]
Express condolences.	R.B., I'm so sorry that you and your family have to go through such a difficult time.
Search for anger.	These events can generate intense anger. Are these feelings that you have had, and if so, where are they directed? [This discussion is central to this case. Initially, the husband may express anger directly at you as the care provider. In response, the follow-up sentence should be:] I can understand why you feel that way. Let us look at the details of the case so that we can try to sort this out. [Review the maneuvers to deliver the baby.]
Describe family dynamics.	Sometimes anger also is directed at a family member because of the outcome. Is this an issue that we should discuss openly? [This difficult component of the conversation may lead nowhere. But in a safe environment, it may allow the husband to express anger at his wife for noncompliance with her diet and insulin therapy as a cause for the fetal macrosomia.]

Conversations to Educate

Points to Cover	The Conversation
Complete the "Feared Factor."	[The remainder of the conversation fulfills the six criteria for the "Feared Factor." The family should be allowed time to explain what they have heard, and issues raised by extended family members should be addressed.]
Document.	[A thorough documentation of the discussion should be entered into the medical record.]

What do I say when, after a bad event, a patient presents me with information she took off the Internet suggesting that a different approach would have resulted in a better outcome?

M.A. is a twenty-four-year-old G2, P1 whose prior pregnancy resulted in a cesarean section at term for a breech presentation. This pregnancy, you have followed her with ultrasounds due to concerns that she is at risk for a placenta acreta because of the prior cesarean section and because the placenta is implanted over the former uterine scar. Preoperatively, she had been properly consented for a cesarean-hysterectomy if needed, due to the risk of hemorrhage. At term, she undergoes a repeat cesarean section with delivery of a healthy newborn son weighing 3300 grams with one- and five-minute Apgar scores of 9 and 10, respectively.

Removal of the placenta produces excessive bleeding that is not easily controlled by compression, uterine artery ligation, or other efforts to control the bleeding at the site of the placental vascular bed. When she has lost 2000 cc of blood, you performed a hysterectomy because of your inability to control the bleeding.

M.A.'s recovery following the hysterectomy is uneventful, albeit emotional. M.A. is from a large family and hoped to have at least five children. While she is in the hospital, you meet with her twice daily and explain the events that led to the decision to do a hysterectomy. The patient is discharged, and a follow-up meeting in two weeks is set to continue the discussion.

When M.A. and her husband come to your office two weeks later, she is very angry and agitated. Once she is in the exam room, she says to you, "You did not tell me the truth. Just look at this!" and she displays an article taken from the Internet in which the role of interventional radiology is described for patients exhibiting excessive bleeding at the time of delivery. The article, though not peer reviewed, describes a new technique in which embolization of the uterine arteries is used to control the bleeding, thereby saving the patient from hysterectomy. You are caught off-guard by this attack and feel vulnerable because you are not aware of this new technique.

You think to yourself:

- What should be my response?
- How honest should I be if I consider admitting that this is a new technology with which I am not familiar?
- How can I explain without looking defensive how new technologies need time for adequate testing?
- How can I continue to maintain the patient's confidence if in fact it appears that I am not practicing modern medicine?

In this scenario, it is understandable that the patient would feel maligned, since she has found information from the Internet that an alternative management might have allowed the preservation of her uterus. A hysterectomy is a devastating event for many women, and the fact that the patient is alive may at first offer little condolence to counter her grief reaction to this loss.

The discussion should start by your expressing sadness that the hysterectomy had to be done and your awareness that she will be grieving not only for the frightening events connected with the surgery but also her loss of fertility. Next, the events leading up to the hysterectomy should be reviewed. At this point, it is appropriate to provide information as to how new technologies are introduced into medicine. Nonmedical people may not realize that new ideas constantly are being generated; some will replace old technologies, and some will be discarded after appropriate testing. In anticipation of this discussion, it may be helpful for you to review some medical discoveries that looked as if they were going to replace old technologies, only later to be abandoned.

At the completion of the discussion, it is important to repeat your feelings of sadness that the hysterectomy had to be done and to state that you appreciate the new information that your patient has provided you. With this new information, which you will read and learn more about, your future patients may benefit from this new technology.

Basic Principles

- Express condolences that the hysterectomy had to be done.
- Review the indications that led to the hysterectomy.
- Express appreciation for the new information the patient has found on the Internet.
- Provide a brief history of the process by which new technologies are introduced in medicine.
- Explain how new technologies need time to mature.
- Give examples of great ideas that later were abandoned.
- Repeat that you are sorry that the hysterectomy had to be done.
- Document the conversation.

Here is how the conversation might go:

Points to Cover	The Conversation
Express your feelings.	M.A., I appreciate the opportunity to meet with you and your husband and to discuss the circumstances around your surgery and the need to perform a cesarean hysterectomy.

Points to Cover	The Conversation
Review the facts.	[A detailed discussion of the sequence of events should be provided in nonmedical terms to explain the decision-making process at the operating table that resulted in the hysterectomy.] I am impressed by the effort that you have made to seek additional information from the Internet, and I thank you for providing that to me. [It may be helpful to inquire whether M.A. has found additional information that should be part of this conversation.]
Discuss how new technology is introduced into medicine.	If the process of medicine does nothing else, it reminds us constantly that it is forever changing. The information that you have provided me represents new technology that is not available in all hospitals. It is likely that this new technology, if proved over time, will in fact change the way in which we respond to acute hemorrhage in the postpartum period.
Give examples of failed technologies.	There are many examples, however, of new ideas that initially were thought to provide a final solution for a medical entity, only to be abandoned later as more rigorous clinical trials proved the new technology to be ineffective. Some of these examples have occurred even within the years that many of us have practiced. The management of a patient with a type of low platelet count, called idiopathic thrombocytopenia purpura, is one such example. In the early 1970s, a cesarean section was carried out routinely because of the fear that the low platelet count in the mother would create a low platelet count in the fetus, thus rendering the baby

Points to Cover	The Conversation
Give examples of failed technologies. (cont.)	at risk for cerebral hemorrhage. Subsequent to that approach, we attempted to sample the scalp blood of the fetus during labor, but that also proved to be technologically difficult. Finally, a thorough analysis showed that the risk to the fetus was far less than the risks from the interventional approaches that we were using to address the problem. We have abandoned any effort to sample the fetal blood for its platelet count and instead now allow labor and vaginal delivery to occur.

Another example is the use of ethanol to stop preterm labor. In the 1970s, we administered intravenous ethanol to pregnant women in preterm labor because of results from studies carried out in animal models indicating that this approach might stop labor. Women were given several liters of 5 percent ethanol intravenously during the first twenty-four hours. You can imagine how terrible these women felt. They became intoxicated as a result of the ethanol exposure. Subsequent to that, we abandoned that approach. |
| **Repeat the importance of the Internet finding.** | Setting those examples aside, however, I do believe that the technologies that you have discovered on the Internet offer us a new direction in the management of postpartum hemorrhage. We must remember that much of the material on the Internet is not accurate or verified. Nonetheless, I will read further on this topic and perhaps will be able to introduce it into my own practice in the future. For that, I thank you for bringing this to my attention. |

132

Points to Cover	The Conversation
Explain the decision.	At the time that I needed to make the decisions regarding your health and the risks of postpartum hemorrhage, I had to rely on the skills that I had available to me in deciding that a hysterectomy was the only way to proceed. I can reassure you that I was fully aware of the effect that this type of surgery would have on your desire for future pregnancies. I hope you will accept my explanation of my actions and the medical care that you received.
Document.	[A thorough documentation of the discussion should be entered into the medical record.]

What do I say when a young colleague calls me announcing that she is leaving medicine? She has experienced her first maternal death under her care and feels unworthy to continue practicing medicine.

You have just settled in for an afternoon of chart work at your office when your receptionist relays a call to you from a young colleague, B.J., whom you knew initially as a resident and now practices with another group. You remember her as very solid as a resident, who always was good with patients and had a good knowledge of the field. Although B.J. now is two years out from her residency, you have been in touch with her on several occasions and continue to be impressed by the care she provides her patients.

The conversation is not what you expected. B.J., obviously distraught, tells you that she is leaving medicine. Taken aback, you inquire why, and then are provided the following answer: B.J. describes managing her patient in labor, a twenty-eight-year-old G1, P0 at term. Labor progression had been slow. When the patient had gotten to 5 centimeters dilated and remained there for one hour, B.J. palpated her uterine contractions and felt that they were adequate. She chose not to place an intrauterine pressure catheter or to augment with Pitocin since she believed that the labor contractions were appropriate, despite failure of cervical dilation. She elected to perform a cesarean section, which was carried out under spinal anesthesia. The surgery was uncomplicated.

After she was sure her postoperative patient was stable, B.J. left the recovery room in order to make additional ward rounds. Within minutes, she heard an overhead page to her and ran to the unit: her patient was undergoing a full resuscitation that ultimately proved unsuccessful. The husband and family, obviously distraught, were brought into another room and with the help of one of her partners, were provided a description of the labor, the surgery, and the woman's sudden death.

In the discussion with the family, a number of possible explanations were raised, including pulmonary embolism or amniotic fluid embolism. The need for an autopsy was raised. The family declined the autopsy, even though they were approached a second time within the next two hours. After several hours, the family departed to make funeral arrangements and to figure how to raise the newborn.

B.J. was overwhelmed by the knowledge that this was the first patient she had cared for directly who had died. She felt a terrible sense of responsibility. Should she have waited longer before performing the cesarean section? Should she have stayed with the patient longer in the postoperative period? Was there any warning of the impending death that she missed? Was she a bad person for somehow causing this event? How could the family ever have faith in her again after this?

In her call to you, she concludes that she is not worthy to practice medicine, that somehow she should have been able to do something that would have resulted in a different outcome. She asserts that it would be better if she leaves medicine completely and therefore leaves the care of patients to others more capable of carrying this responsibility.

You console B.J. by expressing your understanding of her feelings, and in the back of your mind you reflect back on your own similar experiences. You arrange to meet with her later that afternoon.

In anticipation of the meeting, you ask yourself these questions:

- How can I discuss my feelings regarding the management of her patient, elements of which I may not have agreed with, and yet still keep the focus on her abrupt decision to leave medicine?
- How can I reassure her that she still is a valued contributor to medicine?
- How can I help her as she interacts with the family?

That evening, you initiate a conversation with B.J. by acknowledging the intense emotions that are generated within a care provider when the first patient dies under his or her care. You even may admit that it brings strong feelings back from similar experiences you had as a young care provider. Having made that admission, you provide a platform for the remainder of this discussion by reaffirming that the training that B.J. received as a resident was high quality and now allows her to provide her patients an equally high level of medicine.

You state that patients whom B.J. has cared for since graduating from the residency applaud her skills and describe her as a good doctor. With these comments as a base, it is reasonable to review what would be lost if B.J. chose to leave medicine because of this event. You point out that medicine is an art form more than a science. You comment that medicine simply is people working with other people using the resources at hand. You also note that sometimes adverse medical events occur, even under the watchful eye of the most skilled practitioner. You query B.J. as to what benefit would be achieved by her leaving medicine. Would her patients find other physicians as committed as she to their care? And you ask B.J. whether she believes that the process of medical care always must result in a "win" or if patients seek care from a doctor who will commit to engineering that process with the hope of a good outcome.

Allowing B.J. to reflect on her role as a physician to provide care to a patient and family, even if an adverse event occurs and even if it is independent of her care, reinforces the idea that medical care truly is a process, not merely an end point. B.J. may reconsider her decision if she is challenged by questions regarding the fate of her other patients if she runs

Conversations to Educate

away from this challenge. When emotions are involved, it is important to compartmentalize them. The question of whether B.J. should have allowed labor to continue longer or whether she should have stayed with her patient after the surgery can be discussed separately from reviewing the impact of the death on B.J.'s impressions of her own integrity. Despite this adverse event, reinforcement that she is a good physician who is recognized by her patients for her attentiveness and compassion should encourage B.J. to develop a more positive attitude about herself.

If, after such a discussion, your young colleague still is unwilling to reconsider her decision, other steps may be needed. Professional counseling to help her cope with the feelings of loss is one approach. With her concurrence, asking a colleague to mentor her for a period of time is another. Finally, suggesting that she take some time off may allow her to reconsider the events and rebuild her self-worth.

Examples of statements you thought you stated one way, yet were interpreted by your patient to mean something else

Fundamental to good medical care is the ability of the care provider and patient to discuss complex issues on a common level where what the care provider says is interpreted accurately by the patient, who then can ask questions of the care provider.

In many ways, good communication is the backbone of good medical care. But medical care brings two individuals to the conversation table whose backgrounds often are disparate. The care provider is knowledgeable in medical terminology and inserts that understanding into common dialogue. The patient may be equally professional in his or her own field, but may not grasp the subtleties of the messages being transmitted during such a dialogue. Few care providers at the completion of a discussion with the patient ask the patient to recite back what he or she interpreted. When they do, they are often astonished to realize how little communication actually has transpired: in a discussion covering fifteen or twenty minutes, the patient may be able to recite back only two or three points out of many covered in that discussion.

Following are examples of statements made with good intent by the care provider but may be interpreted incorrectly, thus providing a barrier to future communication and a threat to the relationship between the care provider and the patient:

• "Ms J., I have received the results of the biopsy and it could be cancer." From this statement the care provider is indicating that the test results, while equivocal, may ultimately lead to a diagnosis of cancer. The care provider is preparing the patient for the possibility of this diagnosis. What is missing in this discussion is the opportunity for the care provider to introduce the possibility of a range of diagnoses, starting initially with a noncancer diagnosis, but then moving toward a more ominous diagnosis such as cancer. The same information could be conveyed simply by saying, "Ms. J., we have received the results of the biopsy. The results are still pending, and so even as we discuss the possibilities, we must await a final diagnosis in order to be certain. The diagnosis could be simply cellular changes reflecting inflammation or infection. We must be aware, however, of the fact that other diagnoses, including even cancer, will have to be evaluated." By approaching the test results in this way and providing the wide range of possibilities, the patient is brought into the discussion and continues to listen to the possibilities. If only the possibility of cancer is introduced, it is likely the patient will not hear any other consideration for diagnosis.

• "Mrs. S., we have been following the test results for several days. I suspect that you may already have anticipated what I'm about to say." This statement is made by the care provider with the intention of acknowledging that the patient is intelligent enough to be able to understand the ramifications of the test results. The care provider may be surprised by the negative manner in which the patient reacts to this statement. This is because the care provider is assuming that the patient has already discounted everything but the worst news. This statement also implies that if the patient had become used to the idea of the diagnosis, he or she already would have resolved some fear and anxiety. The patient, however, perceives the statement as insensitive because it does not allow her to process the information leading ultimately to the diagnosis.

• "Mrs. P., we have finished your ultrasound but cannot see all of the baby's spine." This statement, frequently made in ultrasound or radiology laboratories, indicates that the sonographer or physician was unable to obtain a clear view of the fetal spine due to the fetal position. It is understandable that the patient might conclude that her baby is malformed.

CHAPTER 6

Conversations to Improve Quality of Care

How do I present bad news when there is a language barrier?

You are asked to see a Ukrainian woman who presents at thirty weeks' gestation. She has been seen only twice before in your practice and speaks no English. Her sister, who does speak English, is accompanying her on this clinic visit to translate. In the ultrasound laboratory, no fetal heart tones are detected. She is admitted to labor and delivery, where induction with Pitocin produces a rapid delivery. Although her sister accompanies her throughout the process, your patient remains stoic and nonverbal. Following the delivery, she indicates no interest in having an autopsy. Later that afternoon, you arrange to sit with the patient and her sister.

You ask yourself:

- How do I present the news?
- To whom do I present the information?
- What is the role of the sister as interpreter as opposed to an outside interpreter?
- What explanation should I provide the patient through the interpreter that would be understood?

When conversing with a non-English-speaking patient, there is a style to the discussion that does not exist when the same conversation is carried out between a care provider and patient for which English is her first language. It goes without saying that speaking loudly offers little to improve the communication through the interpreter and should be avoided. One also must be careful not to interpret a patient's head nodding as a signal that she understands the conversation. In many cultures, nodding is a courtesy that implies that the conversation is ongoing, not necessarily that it is understood.

The role of the interpreter in such a session is essential for communicating accurately to the patient, but that role also must be understood clearly by the care provider. It is wise not to use a family member as a substitute interpreter, since there may be conflict of interest or other personal or family agendas that influence the conversation and that you as the care provider would not recognize.

When speaking to a patient through an interpreter, direct comments at the patient. The fact that the patient is looking at the interpreter should not change this orientation of the conversation. The discussion should follow the format of the "Feared Factor." The style of the conversation, however, may be different. Long sentences should be replaced by short sentences. The need to express medical terms in simple nonmedical language is even more important than in the usual care provider–patient conversation. Encouraging the patient through the interpreter to address back to you her understanding of the conversation is essential. Pausing between topic items clarifies groups of ideas. At the completion of the discussion, indicate how the patient could obtain more information on the issues discussed once she has returned home in case her family members have questions. Then document the conversation.

Basic Principles

- Speak directly to the patient, not to the interpreter.

- Express sympathy and indicate (if appropriate) that the outcome was not because of something the patient did.

What Do I Say?

- Use short sentences.
- If long sentences are required, pause at the end of phrases so that the interpreter can communicate your thoughts accurately.
- Pause between topic items in case the patient wants to express to the interpreter a question regarding your comments.
- At the end of each topic covered, ask (through the interpreter) the patient to relay back to you what she perceives that you said to her.
- At the completion of the conversation, provide information through the interpreter as to how the patient can obtain more information if additional questions arise once she returns home.
- Document the conversation.

Here is how the conversation provided through an interpreter might go:

Points to Cover	The Conversation
Express your feelings.	Mrs. G., I am sorry about the death of your baby. Your sadness is made even greater because you are not in your native country and I am unable to speak your language. [Pause for interpreter.]
Describe the facts.	From what I know of your pregnancy, we can be comforted by the knowledge that you did nothing yourself that contributed to your baby's death. It is very sad when a baby dies. It is even sadder when a parent feels responsible for the death. [Pause for interpreter.] I am aware that you did not want to have an autopsy for your baby. This is a very personal choice. At delivery, the appearance of your baby provided us no information as to why your baby died. However, because your baby appeared normal, it is likely that your baby died by pinching its umbilical cord, which brings oxygen and food to a baby when it is inside the uterus. [Pause for interpreter.]

Points to Cover	The Conversation
Review discussions about burial and availability of support systems.	[At this point, the conversation, provided in short segments, might explore how the family might dispose of the baby's body and what type of support the woman has within her community as she struggles to make sense of her baby's death. Identifying important support people in her family may be even more important when language barrier complicates the counseling session than when English is the spoken language.]
Have the issues recited back to you through the interpreter.	Mrs. G., we are now at the end of our counseling session. I would like you to explain to the interpreter what your understanding is of my comments so that I can be sure that we have communicated accurately. [A conversation should follow between the woman and the interpreter to document that the information was provided. Finally, the woman should be provided information as to whom she or other family members can call if additional questions surface when she returns home and attempts to communicate the information provided during the counseling session to her family members.]
Document.	[After the conversation, document the details of the discussion, the individuals who attended, the interpreter and company she is hired by, the tone of the conversation, and the next stages of care.]

Should I ever deliver bad news over the telephone or by e-mail?

L.G. is a thirty-eight-year-old G1, P0. She lives with her husband in a small town approximately 150 miles from the regional perinatal center. After appropriate genetic counseling, she chooses to have an amniocentesis carried out at the perinatal center. Two weeks later, the genetics department at the regional perinatal center learns that L.G.'s fetus has Down syndrome. The senior genetic counselor calls L.G.'s obstetrician, who lives in the next town approximately twenty miles away to inform her of the findings. L.G.'s physician, now armed with this information, must decide how this is best given to L.G.

The physician asks:

- Should L.G. be told over the telephone?
- If L.G. is told to come into the office, will this communicate clearly that the results are bad?
- How can a care provider be sure that the information has been received accurately?

Due to geographic constraints, sometimes bad news must be transmitted to a patient who does not reside in the immediate area of the care provider's facility. As a general principle, bad news should never be conveyed over the telephone. That said, circumstances sometimes force the need for the care provider to deliver information over the telephone even if it is against his or her better judgment. The obvious preferred approach is to contact the patient and arrange for her to come into the office, where the information can be delivered. With some techniques or laboratory tests, it is not surprising that a patient immediately would recognize the threatening nature of the conversation. In this situation, the patient likely would assume that if the results were normal, this information could be given over the telephone. Why, then, would she need to come into the office merely to discuss normal results?

Because the telephone call may escalate into a conversation even as the care provider is attempting to avoid it, the care provider who makes the call should be the one most knowledgeable about the results and be prepared to answer all of the questions likely to be generated by the conversation. If a full disclosure needs to be given over the telephone, the care provider should have left ample time for the discussion. In that discussion, the care provider may wish to inquire if the patient understands the facts. It may be prudent to defer that approach, replacing it with a visit to your office or a follow-up telephone call in one or two days. By then, the patient will have had the time to absorb the news and will be better prepared to indicate her level of understanding. She also will be better positioned to ask questions that might have eluded her during the first telephone call. The care provider should inquire as to family support immediately available to the patient who has been given bad news over the telephone.

E-mail offers an equal challenge to good communication. Advocated as a rapid form of communication, it risks conveying incomplete ideas in favor of brevity. Unlike a formal face-to-face conference, where the ideal conversation should have been scripted mentally by the care provider before the meeting, messages sent by e-mail lack human elements of body language, facial gestures, or personal warmth. The facts may be communicated in a timely way, but the method of communication is personally flat.

Most good communicators recognize that an important part of the message is the input that the communicator receives during the conversation. Does the patient understand what I am saying? Am I describing the details too quickly? Will questions the patient asks during the conversation aid me in directing the discussion in a way that is more understandable to the patient? Will our personal interactions during our conversation aid in dispensing misconceptions and suspicion? Negative answers to these questions may be the major limitations of using e-mail to convey bad news.

Basic Principles

- If possible, never deliver bad news over the telephone or by e-mail.
- If a telephone conversation is necessary, allow ample time for the conversation to proceed in an unhurried way.
- Be certain that you understand all aspects of the issue and can answer all of the questions that might be generated.
- Inquire about support people in the house or neighborhood.
- During a follow-up telephone call, ask that the patient describe back the issues that have been discussed to ensure that there was clarity in the communication.

- If e-mail must be used, define a specific time when the patient should get back to you with responses and questions.
- Document the entire conversation in the medical record.

Here is how the conversation might go:

Points to Cover	The Conversation
Be careful with the introduction.	[The telephone rings, and Mrs. L.G. answers it.] Mrs. L.G., this is Dr. S. I am calling regarding the genetic amniocentesis that you had two weeks ago. In general, we like to sit with each family to discuss the results, and I was wondering if you would be able to come to the office this afternoon or tomorrow to review these results. [At this point, the patient may say yes, not concluding that bad results have been encountered. However, the patient also may launch into an inquiry as to what the results are, since, if they were normal, there should be no problem in giving them over the phone. In this case, Mrs. L.G. does just that.]
Deliver the news concisely.	Mrs. L.G., unfortunately, the results are not normal. It appears that the results of the amniocentesis indicate that your baby has Down syndrome. Are you familiar with the term *Down syndrome?* [Mrs. L.G. may express great concern or even terror, and a brief period may need to lapse before she is able to regain her composure.]
Ask to include a support person.	Mrs. L.G., is your husband available, perhaps to listen to this conversation on another line?
Describe the information in simple terms.	[After Mr. L.G. is on the telephone, the doctor continues:] Down syndrome is . . . [Keep the conversation concise. A lengthier discussion should occur in the follow-up conversation.]

Points to Cover	The Conversation
Apologize for using the telephone for this conversation.	Mr. and Mrs. L.G., let me repeat, I am sorry that we have had to get into this conversation over the telephone, as I know there are many questions that you have.
Offer to follow up in person that day if possible.	I do believe that it is important for you to come to my office today or tomorrow, because there are many issues that still need to be dealt with, and I can take you through them in a step-by-step manner. It is also important for you to be aware of the many community services available to families whose children have Down syndrome. This would be a meaningful discussion, and I think it would assist you as you begin to factor the information I have provided into your family setting.
Ask about community support services.	Are there other family members or friends in your community who can provide assistance to you and who may wish to come with you to the office so that they too can hear about the issues and some of the community services that are available?
Inform your receptionist of the proposed office visit.	[The office receptionist should be informed that when Mrs. L.G. and her husband come into the waiting area, they should be directed through and into a separate room and not be required to sit in the waiting area along with other pregnant patients.]
Document.	[A thorough documentation of the discussion should be entered into the medical record.]

How should I use past experiences the patient has encountered as a guide for how she will react and manage bad news?

An important component of deciphering how a patient is responding to a crisis is to discuss how he or she has dealt with past crises. The conversation may begin with a question: "Have you ever faced similar events in the past, and, if so, how have you dealt with them?" If the patient replies that she has never had anything like this happen before in her life, pursuing this line of discussion may offer little value. It may however provide a baseline of emotional challenges that she has encountered previously and coping skills for dealing with the situation she is facing now. It then may be appropriate to ask how, if she has encountered events like this in the past, she anticipates approaching this problem.

If the discussion is approached in this manner, she may provide insight into past losses, such as losing a job, divorce, death of a loved one, or episodes of depression, which can be a starting point for dealing with the situation. Practical questions provide valuable information:

"From whom have you sought help during difficult times?"

"With whom do you commonly speak about difficult issues in your life?"

"Why have you chosen these individuals, and what benefit have they provided?"

"Are these same individuals available now? Do you think they can provide similar support during this crisis?"

In taking such a history, the questioner must ask also whether, in the past, difficult times have prompted the individual to believe that life was not worth living or, worse, that she might consider killing herself because life seemed worthless. This question, if posed in a compassionate way, most likely will be answered with a convincing "no" and need not be pursued. If, however, she answers yes to this line of questioning, these issues must be pursued in order to determine if the individual would view the current crisis also as a reason to revisit those thoughts of life not worth living.

How should I use religion as a base for constructing a path of recovery?

In an effort to establish the behavioral base on which a patient will respond to this moment of crisis, it is important to consider other avenues of support. For some families, religion offers that type of support.

A useful question is, "Are you a religious person? If so, do you feel that religion provides you some answers as to why your loss occurred?" If she answers, "No, I am not a religious person," pursuing this line of questioning may not offer benefit. However, imagine the following response: "Yes, I am a deeply religious person, and I believe that it is God's will that this outcome occurred." This response may allow you a second line of questioning: "If you believe that it is God's will, what role do you feel that your care providers have in this process?" The answer may be, "It is God's will and not that of the care providers to decide the outcome of my baby." Or you may find that the response is, "God guides the care provider's hands and thoughts in helping me and my family during this time of great tragedy."

By examining such important pillars in life as religion, you may identify the support systems to pursue in future questioning or future visits.

How should I document in the chart?

Documenting accurately the care or advice that a care provider provides patients has several purposes. First and foremost, it serves as a vehicle to communicate the type of care that has been provided and the thought process behind that care when, at a subsequent visit or subsequent treatment, this information becomes part of the continuum of care that the patient received. To this end, it also serves as a record for other care providers who may intervene in the meantime and wish to maintain a certain level of care dictated by the initial documentation. Because of the importance of good documentation, the notations placed in the record should be thoughtful, clearly written, and meaningful to both the writer of the document and other care providers who may read that documentation.

Clear documentation serves other purposes as well. It is possible that every physician will be sued eventually. Documentation in the outpatient and inpatient records serves as protection for the care provider when, years later, the care is reconstructed in a court of law and questions regarding the care are generated. Documentation as a contemporary tool of communication and as an asset when one's level of care has been challenged in a court of law are two important reasons why successful care providers consistently produce accurate documentation.

Unlike hospital-based health professionals for whom there is one chart only for documenting the unanticipated outcome discussion with patients, physicians often dictate or write a note in office-based records about aspects of the discussion that took place outside the hospital. Indeed, this is likely if the patient needs two or more "sit-down" sessions with the doctor or he or she responds to a series of follow-up questions posed by the patient in a telephone conversation.

Many health care facilities have developed protocols or processes for documenting discussions about unanticipated outcomes. Some encourage more succinct documentation practices, and others promote a more detailed notation. Some frown on the idea of documenting the dialogue in the medical record out of concern that it may be used against the facility in the event that a lawsuit arises from the occurrence. Those who take this perspective may require that the caregiver write in the progress notes, "Outcome discussion transpired with patient and family members [names inserted here]." The note then is signed and dated. A fuller explanation of the event may then be dictated or written in some other institutional document that is geared toward peer review, process improvement, or, if litigation is contemplated, risk management.

Office-based records do not tend to follow this approach. Indeed, many practices do not have a formal policy on how to document the discussion of an adverse event. What is written may be left to the discretion of an individual doctor.

As experience has grown with unanticipated outcome disclosures, a danger exists if there is a discrepancy between notations in the office-based record and hospital documentation. If discoverable and admissible in court, the discrepancy could be used to the detriment of the facility and caregivers. It could be used to challenge the credibility of the outcomes discussion, impeach witnesses, or as evidence of a breach of a standard of care. The idea that "someone is trying to cover his tracks" might be reflected in such a documentation discrepancy.

There are steps that can be taken to avoid such difficulties. One is to encourage the hospital and the medical staff to develop a consistent documentation style. Such an initiative might be driven by medical staff leadership in the institution. Recognizing that there will be a need for flexibility and format, the goal should be a consistent approach to what is documented and how it is stated in writing. If the hospital uses paper records and the office is paperless, the media may be different, but the essential notation elements should be transparent from one venue to another.

Another possibility is to design one approach that can be used in either setting, perhaps as a template. If a decision is made to use one tool or template, it should be reviewed by legal counsel, risk management, and, in the hospital setting, the forms committee.

A third approach is to develop one template that serves the fundamental needs of both the health care facility and the physician. Additional documentation opportunity may be granted for the office-based practice so that the physician can document evening and off-hour telephone calls with the patient and follow-up items that come up as a result of the basic disclosure discussion.

Whatever methodology is used, a key step is to teach health professionals how to document the disclosure discussion. Some approaches are better than others in documenting such conversations. The goal, however, should be to document well in the midst of a stressful obstetric case. The documentation should be clear, concise, and factually based.

Following are the elements of good documentation:

• *Date and time every note.* Picture the twenty-four-year-old G1, P0 admitted at thirty-three weeks' gestation with chronic hypertension and superimposed preeclampsia. The patient stabilizes at bed rest until early in the morning hours of the second day of hospitalization, when the nurse calls you out of the sleeproom to see the patient because of her progressively rising blood pressures and a headache. You see the patient and in your note indicate the day of the visit but do not write down the time. You see the patient again at 6:00 A.M., but because you are making brief rounds before you go to the office, you do not write a note.

As you arrived at the office at 7:30 A.M., your beeper goes off and you learn that your patient is seizing. You return quickly to the hospital and provide appropriate care by delivering the patient by cesarean section. The baby does not do well, despite appropriate neonatal support, and exhibits seizure activity in the newborn period. You counsel the family regarding the dangers of eclampsia and assume that the family is satisfied with the answers that you have provided.

Five years later, this patient sues you, and the discussion in court regarding patient care focuses on the lack of documentation. You claim that you saw the patient shortly before she seized and at that visit she exhibited stable vital signs. Had an accurate note been placed in the records indicating the day *and* time, the information available at that 6:00 A.M. visit would have been helpful in defending the fact that you did not decide to deliver the patient by cesarean section at that time. Lacking that information, you are vulnerable to the criticism that you abandoned the patient after her condition merited closer observation than you had provided and therefore you were at fault.

• *Write legibly.* This seems like a simple statement but cannot be emphasized enough. Picture this scenario: your twenty-two-year-old G1, P0 at twenty-two weeks' gestation ruptures her membranes and presents without labor in your triage area. After adequate counseling and with the understanding that this is a nonviable state, the patient elects to be induced into labor to avoid the possibility that her newborn will be resuscitated vigorously and either die after an extended period or survive with major disabilities. The notation you write in the record is difficult to decipher, even as you have indicated that no heroic measures will be made at the time of the delivery. The patient responds to the Pitocin, but your partner is on that night. Because she cannot read your writing, there is some confusion as to whether this is a twenty-two-week or a twenty-six-week gestation. At the delivery, an uninformed pediatrician is asked to evaluate the newborn quickly and mistakenly concludes that the newborn should be resuscitated. He too cannot decipher your note. Vigorous resuscitation ensues; the newborn, subsequently judged to be twenty-three weeks' gestation, is placed on a ventilator and later develops cerebral palsy accompanied by mental retardation. Had a clear note been written detailing the plans for management and the patient's desires, the mix-up in management would have been eliminated, and a lawsuit would also have been avoided.

• *Do not insert your own personal opinions of another care provider or patient in the records.* This is an important principle. Imagine that you are cross-covering for another private practice. In the records, you read the note of a care provider who indicates that his patient, R.J., who has lost a previous pregnancy at sixteen weeks' gestation, should be evaluated carefully for circlage placement in this current pregnancy. You are in the hospital and covering over the weekend when the patient calls complaining of pelvic pressure at fifteen weeks' gestation. At the first call, you have the patient come into triage, but a vaginal examination fails to reveal any dilation of the cervix. The patient returns home and two hours later calls back again. At this time, you merely reassure her that nothing is wrong. You write in the records that the patient obviously is anxious and overwrought, but will do fine. The patient calls later that day, and you reassure her again. This time, you write in the record that the patient is overly anxious, that her physician probably overreacted, and that the patient probably is somewhat neurotic from her past experiences. You also write that the patient does not seem very intelligent and that a "lack of gray matter" may really be her problem. She is told not to bother you unless there's something really significant to complain about.

Ninety minutes later, she returns to triage 5 centimeters dilated and delivers within an hour. In the courts years later, your note is magnified such that the letters are three feet high. All of the jury members can see the statements that you entered into the record clearly and, more important, can sense the mood in which you entered those statements. It is understandable that some patients may seek excessive care for conditions that do not merit that degree of care. Expressing anger in a permanent record, however, can lead only to misperceptions of the intent of the care provider to provide quality care. Keeping personal statements out of the records is fundamental to good record keeping.

• *Never alter the chart.* Picture this scenario: your twenty-year-old G1, P0 is admitted with mild preeclampsia at thirty-seven weeks' gestation. In the morning, you write a note in the record indicating that you will most likely consider an induction the next day. Later that afternoon, the family approaches you in the hall worried; their daughter seems more listless and appears somewhat difficult to arouse. Your day has been long, and you are ready to get home. You reassure the family that you saw the daughter earlier in the day and you are sure that she is doing fine. You also indicate that when she is seen the next day, a lengthier discussion regarding induction will occur. That evening, your patient seizes and ends up in the adult intensive care unit. She has a stormy course and is left with neurologic deficit. Two days after the seizure, you enter a small note after your daytime note written in the morning that the patient seized. You indicate your concern for the patient because of her changing mental state and the possibility that you may have to intervene possibly even that night.

Several years later in a court of law, you attempt to defend the statements in the record. The family clearly remembers a different scenario, which they describe in their testimony. You lose the case because the jury does not believe that you made your notations at the time you indicated in the records.

Good documentation is the best friend of a care provider. It serves as a contemporary communication and as protection years later in a lawsuit when the details of patient management cannot be remembered accurately. Establishing a correct date and time, documenting contemporaneously, documenting objectively and accurately, writing legibly, avoiding emotional statements or statements made out of anger, and avoiding criticism of others make for a valuable communication.

How do I arrange the furniture in my office for effective counseling?

Offices can be arranged to improve the communication between care provider and patient. It is recognized that different patients require different environments in order that effective communication can occur. Three of these settings are shown in Figure 6.1.

Figure 6.1A shows what might be referred to as an authoritarian environment. In this arrangement, the physician sits behind a large desk and the patient sits on the other side. The physician is dressed in a white coat as an authoritative figure and is surrounded by textbooks and other literature as evidence of his education. In this setting, the care provider communicates information from a position of power and authority, and the patient receives this information in a somewhat passive and subordinate position.

Some patients may interpret this as a defensive posture; they see the care provider as needing to be surrounded by evidence of his education and position and thus chooses to be separated physically from the patient by a large desk. Other patients may seek this type of environment as reassurance of the provider's education and authority and may appreciate this traditional style of medicine.

In Figure 6.1B, in what might be called the professional environment, the care provider sits across a smaller table, thereby removing the physical obstacle of the large desk. The setting is no longer surrounded by books and other evidence of academic achievement. This modification of the authoritarian environment nevertheless maintains certain components of it. Although this setting is less formal, the care provider still wears the white coat, which sends an authoritative message. Some patients prefer, or even expect, this balance of authority and informality.

In Figure 6.1C, the most informal setting shown here, the care provider has removed his medical coat, there is no physical barrier between him and the patient, and the books have been replaced by a nonmedical setting. This informal room arrangement establishes a level of trust in which care provider and care recipient are on the same level, even as the patient is there to receive care and the care provider is there to provide care. This

154

Figure 6.1. Office Settings for Counseling.
(A) The Authoritarian Environment. (B) The Professional
Environment. (C) The Informal Setting.

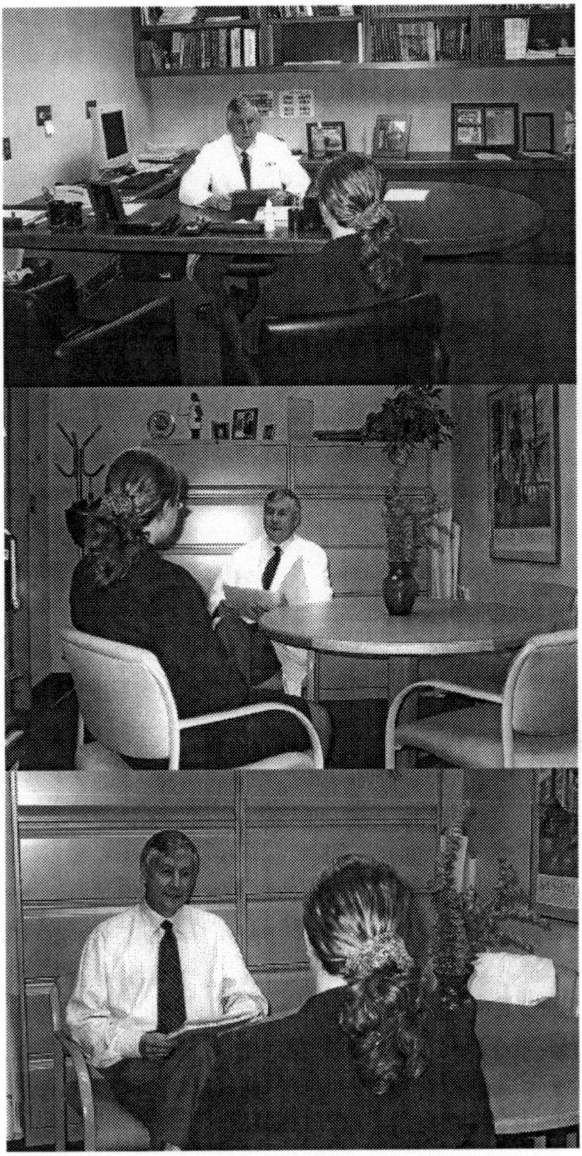

(A)

(B)

(C)

arrangement has the advantage of removing any of the physical barriers to communication. Some may criticize its informal atmosphere. Nonetheless, in this environment, there is the optimal opportunity for exchange of ideas on a common level between care provider and care recipient.

Each setting in Figure 6.1 projects a different style of communication. All three settings are acceptable room arrangements for counseling patients, but each setting appeals to a different type of patient. Not all care providers realize that. It is not typical for most care providers to take time to analyze their own environment. By doing so, they may gain insight into methods for improving communication with their patients.

How can I be a more effective communicator on ward rounds?

How a patient is approached when ward rounds are being made influences his or her reaction to the care provider. Imagine this scenario: your patient has gone through a labor that resulted in a cesarean section for cephalopelvic disproportion. A partner in your practice rounded on the patient the next day because you were unavailable. You round on day two. As you enter her room, you have one of two approaches. In the first you say, "Hi, Mrs. J., you look great considering the fact that you have gone through surgery and are only two days out. How well you are doing may even surprise you." Then the conversation proceeds to address how she is doing and some of the steps that are being taken: removal of the Foley catheter, a change in the intravenous administration of fluids, and advancement of diet. In the second approach, you say as you enter the room, "Mrs. J., how are you feeling?" Your face has no expression, and the message it conveys to the patient is, *I anticipate that you must feel bad, because you are only two days out from surgery.*

The first approach understandably can be overdone. It is inappropriate to tell a patient who is one day out from surgery that she looks fabulous or use some other descriptor that makes no sense. A better choice is to make statements implying that she will recover and that her care providers feel good about the progress that she is making. This sends an important message to the patient that she will recover and that there are no issues to be

What Do I Say?

addressed overtly or covertly. The second approach conveys a different message: that patients in a hospital are ill. Although that may be the case in general, no patient wants to remain ill. By expressing through facial expression or body language one's doubt that the patient will improve, the care provider establishes a negative tone and in effect reduces the patient's hope for recovery.

The suggestion that following an adverse event, the physician should find time in the hospital to meet with the family may be controversial. Statements such as, "I do not have time on hospital rounds to sit with a patient to engage in such a discussion," seem shortsighted. If that is followed by, "I am a busy physician and have many other commitments this morning as well," that sentiment overlooks one point: time not taken now to engage the patient in a meaningful discussion regarding an adverse event may seem insignificant when that individual subsequently must spend weeks in a court of law because a malpractice case emerged from this same adverse event.

To physicians who persist in their opposition to this concept, we offer the *ten-minute chat*. During the patient's hospitalization, the physician should find the time to sit at the bedside for ten minutes to discuss the patient's medical care and the outcome of her baby. That ten minutes should be devoted exclusively to the events and not simply a social conversation. This ten minutes, which can be exhausting for the care provider, establishes the foundation for further conversation and therefore plays an important role in the patient's overall care. We believe that the ten-minute chat is a fundamental part of the overall care that all patients deserve who have experienced an adverse obstetric outcome.

What is the proper way to place a patient in an examination room before being seen by a physician or nurse practitioner? How should that care provider address the patient on entering the room for the first time?

As a general principle, no patient should be greeted for the first time in an examination room in a partially dressed or draped position. This approach generates a feeling of vulnerability. Perhaps introduced for office efficiency, this practice puts the patient in a dependent role and compromises the initial conversation that otherwise would be carried out by two adults of equal status.

The patient should be escorted to the examination room fully clothed and permitted to sit in a chair. When the care provider enters, he or she should sit down and address the patient by the patient's official title, including last name. The patient most likely will request that an alternative identifier be used. It is inappropriate for a care provider who seeks to be addressed as Dr. _____ to say to the patient, "Well, Julie, . . ." (if this patient is of comparable age or even older than the care provider). Even patients younger than the care provider initially should be addressed in an appropriate way. Most patients will say, "Please call me Betty instead of Ms. Smith." This initial acknowledgment of the patient's status in the nonmedical world exhibits consideration and respect in the medical setting.

Cleanliness is as important in the outpatient setting as in the inpatient setting. As a courtesy to each patient, the care provider should wash his or her hands in view of the patient before the examination begins. This act communicates the message that the patient is not being touched by a care provider whose hands have not been washed between patients.

After the initial introductions and a history are taken, the care provider should step out while the patient is draped properly by a chaperon for the examination. Following the examination, it is appropriate for the care provider again to step out so that the patient can dress. The final discussion should be carried out with the patient sitting in a chair fully clothed and at the same level as the care provider.

This sequence of maneuvers demonstrates respect by the care provider for the patient and encourages effective communication.

CHAPTER 7

Where Do We Go from Here?

C an a physician avert a lawsuit with a proper consent to obstetric services, disclosure of outcomes, and documenting what was said to the patient about an adverse event? No one can guarantee that these will avoid litigation, but they can go a long way toward minimizing problems.

Consent and disclosure are communication tools that can help channel fear, anxiety, and anger. The human touch of saying, "I am sorry," may deter an otherwise hostile person from proceeding with litigation. Getting the problem on the table rather than bottling it up can both deflect a lawsuit and help health care professionals learn how to communicate effectively with patients.

The reality is that a patient who is disposed to filing a lawsuit will do so. No amount of apologies, expressions of regret, or even the human touch will deter such individuals from proceeding with a lawsuit. Like those who accept the information imparted about an unanticipated outcome or adverse event, litigious individuals deserve disclosure about a treatment outcome. When done well, the disclosure of unanticipated outcomes or adverse events may help to put the situation in perspective to lessen recourse to litigation.

Learning what to say is an important tool for all health care professionals. It requires training, tact, skill, and a basic understanding of people. However, learning what to say is but part of a larger context involving consent, communications between caregivers and patients, and patient safety.

Those who see disclosure as an issue of passing interest do not fully appreciate the degree of distrust and dissatisfaction exhibited by patients and their families. Caregivers who persist in viewing consent as a piece of paper are equally incorrect. The consent process sets the stage for the caregiver-patient relationship. It also serves as a powerful, and inexpensive, tool for finding out what is important to the patient and what will or will not work in terms of diagnostic and treatment recommendations. The process enables the caregiver to gauge and adjust expectations of care. Not only does it help to avert misunderstandings, it can help the needless expenditure of health care dollars on tests or treatment that the patient does not want to receive or that may pose serious risk.

Traditionally, caregivers have not been the beneficiaries of copious amounts of education on effective communication. It is a skill that has been learned or modeled on the behaviors of mentors and senior professionals. Some believe that this skill cannot be learned. This is a myth. Even the most reticent health care professional can learn the fundamentals.

In an ideal world, health care professionals would receive regular training on best practices of interpersonal communications. As the case studies in this book show, they would learn how to communicate with other health care professionals and with patients. They would learn what physical signals to look for in the midst of a difficult discussion with a patient or a patient's family. And they would know when to refrain from having challenging conversations.

In the real world, adverse events and unanticipated outcomes take place when such situations are least expected. They are a shock to the system and to the psyche. "Why me?" is the question that reverberates in the minds of the caregiver and the patient. The shock can be numbing, reducing the ability of the caregiver to ask important questions or provide salient answers. Patients may perceive the explanation as inadequate or an effort to hide the truth.

Rather than take the chance of misunderstandings or engendering misperceptions, a better approach is to script the disclosure. Rather than providing a stiff or wooden presentation to the patient, it can serve as a prompt for the caregiver so that key points are not overlooked in what may be a very emotional time for all concerned. The examples provided in this book reiterate this point.

The discussion must be documented to provide a record of the transaction so that in the future, there is a way to validate that it took place. It may prove instrumental in litigation, a regulatory inquiry, or a peer review proceeding.

The laws of each jurisdiction differ, and so do the uses of the documentation by health care facilities, so there is no single right way to document the discussion. Instead, the documentation must fit the needs of the health care organization, including the projected uses of the documentation.

Much can be said for having a policy and procedure on disclosure. Depending on the content, it can address everything from who should speak with the patient and family to management of difficult choices. The American Society for Healthcare Risk Management white paper on disclosure, *Perspective on Disclosure of Unanticipated Outcomes Information,* provides some useful suggestions for such a policy and procedure, and some health care organizations have developed their own based on this set of suggestions.[1]

We suggest that a model policy and procedure on disclosure of adverse and unanticipated outcomes of care should have the following components:

- Policy statement and objectives
- Procedures
- Lexicon of terms
- Time frames for disclosure of information
- Location or settings for discussion
- Permission for others to participate in the discussion
- Accommodation for hearing, linguistic, cultural, or sight impairment
- Provision of support services for patient or family
- Provision of support services for health care professional
- Provision for continuing discussion

- Reporting findings to patient or family
- Documentation requirements

  Names and relationships of attendees

  Time, date, and location of discussion

  Factual summary of disclosure

  Factual summary of discussion

  Recordation of e-mail discussions with patient and family

  Recordation of telephonic discussions with patient and family

  Storage of documentation

  Access to documentation

  Retention of documentation
- Documentation training
- Management of multiple reporting responsibilities stemming from the same adverse event or unanticipated outcomes of care

  QIO reports or response to QIO inquiries

  Formal patient grievance under the conditions of participation in Medicare and Medicaid for hospitals

  State agency reporting or response to state agency inquiries

  Mandatory reporting of abuse, neglect, or public health reporting

  Common Rule adverse event reporting in clinical trials occurrences

  Medical examiner or coroner case reporting

  Centers for Medicare and Medicaid Services (CMS) reporting or responses to CMS inquiries

  Internal investigations

  Root cause analysis
- Management of exceptional cases

  Child abuse

  Elder abuse

Criminal investigations

Therapeutic privilege

Minor requests parents not be informed

Disputes among family members

Staff refused to engage in discussion with patient or family

Request for transcriptionist

Request for audiotape

Request for videotape

Request for participation by legal counsel

Request for information from the media

- Follow-up to investigations: Disclosure to patients and family members
- Orientation programs

New employees

Students

House staff

Medical staff

Employees

Temporary employees

Volunteers

- Demonstrated competencies in disclosure
- In-service updates

Accountable health care organizations and professions strive for a transparent approach to disclosure of adverse events and unanticipated outcomes. Guided by ethical principles, the goal is to provide open and constructive discussions when there is an untoward result from tests or treatment.

"Transparent" does not mean making an admission of culpability or finger-pointing or setting up someone as a scapegoat for a bad result.

Rather, it is about taking ownership that the result was different from that desired or anticipated by all concerned. An acknowledgment and a simple apology is not tantamount to an admission of liability. This understanding must be instilled in those who participate in orientation and in-service education.

By combining the elements of the consent process at the outset and the disclosure strategies described in this book, caregivers can rise to a new level in patient care, geared to better communication and quality outcomes in obstetrics.

NOTES

Chapter One

1. L. T. Kohn, J. M. Corrigan, and M. S. Donaldson (eds.), *To Err Is Human: Building a Safer Health System* (Washington, D.C.: National Academy Press, 1999).
2. Quality Interagency Coordination Task Force, *Doing What Counts for Patient Safety: Federal Actions to Reduce Medical Errors and Their Impact* (Feb. 2000).
3. Agency for Health Care Research and Quality, *Making Health Care Safer: A Critical Analysis of Patient Safety Practices* (July 2001).
4. Agency for Health Care Research and Quality, *Making Health Care Safer.*
5. "Final Summary of Food and Drug Administration (FDA) Action Items—Doing What Counts for Patient Safety: Federal Actions to Reduce Medical Errors and Their Impact," US Food and Drug Administration, CDER, Feb. 27, 2001.
6. *Federal Register,* July 2, 1999, p. 36070.
7. President's Advisory Commission on Consumer Protection and Quality in the Health Care Industry, *Quality First: Better Health Care for All Americans* (Mar. 1998). See also President's Advisory Commission on Consumer Protection and Quality in the Health Care Industry Quality, *Consumers' Rights and Responsibilities* (Nov. 1997), which devotes an entire chapter to the subject of disclosure of information to consumers in order that they are able to make informed decisions regarding health care.
8. President's Advisory Commission, *Quality First.* See also *Federal Register,* July 2, 1999.
9. See Pa. Stat. Ann. 40 sec. 1303.308 (2002); Revised Code of Washington, sec. 70.41.200 (2000). See also Revised Code of Washington, sec. 42.17.310

(2002). For a good discussion on this topic, see M. Chiang, "Promoting Patient Safety: Creating a Workable Reporting System," *Yale Journal on Regulation* 18 (2001): 383.

10. Chiang, "Promoting Patient Safety." See also Kohn, Corrigan, and Donaldson (eds.), *To Err Is Human.*

11. Okla. Revised Stat. Ann.

12. Minn. Stat. Ann. sec. 145.64 (2001).

13. La. Revised Stat. Ann. LSA-R.S. 13:3715.3 (2001).

14. Kohn, Corrigan, and Donaldson (eds.), *To Err Is Human.*

15. Kohn, Corrigan, and Donaldson (eds.), *To Err Is Human,* p. 96.

16. See Jackson v. Power, 743 P.2d 1376 (Alaska 1987); and Simmons v. Tuomey Regional Medical Center, 533 S.E.2d 312 (S.C. 2000).

17. Baptist Memorial Hospital System v. Sampson, 969 S.W.2d 945 (Tex. 1998).

18. For additional resources on the subject, see B. A. Liang, "The Adverse Event of Unaddressed Medical Error: Identifying and Filling the Holes in the Health-Care and Legal Systems," *Journal of Law, Medicine and Ethics* 29 (2001): 346; R. A. Bovbjerg, R. H. Miller, and D. W. Shapiro, "Paths to Reducing Medical Injury: Professional Liability and Discipline vs. Patient Safety—and the Need for a Third Way," *Journal of Law, Medicine and Ethics* 29 (2001): e69; L. L. Leape, D. D. Woods, M. J. Hatlie, et al., "Promoting Patient Safety by Preventing Medical Error," *Journal of the American Medical Association,* Oct. 28, 1998; D. A. Studdert, E. J. Thomas, J. P. Newhouse, et al., "Can the United States Afford a 'No Fault' System of Compensation for Medical Injury?" *Law and Contemporary Problems* 60 (1997): 1; and W. G. Johnson, T. A. Brennan, J. P. Newhouse, et al., "The Economic Consequences of Medical Injuries: Implications for a No-Fault Insurance Plan," *Journal of the American Medical Association,* May 13, 1992, pp. 2487–2492.

19. *The External Review of Hospital Quality: The Role of Accreditation* (July 1999); *The External Review of Hospital Quality: The Role of Medicare Certification* (July 1999); and *The External Review of Hospital Quality: Holding the Reviewers Accountable* (July 1999).

20. Kohn, Corrigan, and Donaldson (eds.), *To Err Is Human.*

21. See Joint Commission on Accreditation of Healthcare Organizations, Sentinel Event Policy and Procedure.

22. See Joint Commission on Accreditation of Healthcare Organizations, Patient Safety Standards, RI.1.2.2.

23. American Society for Healthcare Risk Management, *Perspective on Disclosure of Unanticipated Outcome Information* (Chicago: American Society for Healthcare Risk Management, July 2001).

24. See Minnesota Hospital and Healthcare Partnership, *Communicating Outcomes to Patients* (2002).

25. Joint Commission on Accreditation of Healthcare Organizations, "Speak Up: National Campaign Urges Patients to Join Safety Efforts," press release, Mar. 14, 2002.

26. President's Advisory Commission, *Quality First.*

27. "BRT-Sponsored Initiative Focuses on Patient Safety," press release, Jan. 6, 2000.

28. President's Advisory Commission on Consumer Protection and Quality in the Health Care Industry, *Consumers' Rights and Responsibilities* (Nov. 1997). See also President's Advisory Commission, *Quality First.*

29. See Massachusetts Board of Registration in Medicine Physician Profile System, http://www.docboard.org/ma/df/name.html; New York Professional Misconduct and Physician Discipline, http://www.health.state.ny.us/nysdoh/opmc/main.htm; and Virginia Board of Medicine's Practitioner Information, http://www.vahealthprovider.com.

30. This information can be obtained at www.JCAHO.org.

31. "Communicating with Patients About Unanticipated Outcomes," *Norcal Claims Rx,* Sept. 2001. See also Midwest Mutual Insurance Company, *Written Guidance on How to Manage Adverse Outcomes for Physicians* (Midwest Mutual Insurance Company, 2001).

32. A. Witman, D. Park, and S. Hardin, "How Do Patients Want Physicians to Handle Mistakes? A Survey of Internal Medicine Patients in an Academic Setting," *Archives of Internal Medicine* 156 (1996): 2565–2569. See also S. Kraman and G. Hamm, "Risk Management: Extreme Honesty May Be the Best Policy," *Annals of Internal Medicine* 963 (1999): 131.

33. Kraman and Hamm, "Risk Management." See also "Honesty Best Policy?" *Forum* (Feb. 2000).

34. 28 U.S.C. sec. 1346(b).

35. See Minnesota Alliance for Patient Safety, *Call to Action: Roles and Responsibilities for Assuring Patient Safety* (2001).

36. See *Strategies for Leadership: An Organizational Approach to Patient Safety,* VHA (2002).

37. Liang, "The Adverse Event of Unaddressed Medical Error"; Bovbjerg, Miller, and Shapiro, "Paths to Reducing Medical Injury."

38. For a discussion of the topic, see Liang, "The Adverse Event of Unaddressed Medical Error"; *Making Health Care Safer: A Critical Analysis of Patient Safety Practices* (Agency for Health Care Research and Quality, July 2001); Kohn, Corrigan, and Donaldson (eds.), *To Err Is Human;* and F. A. Rozovsky, J. Roosevelt, and K. A. Chaurette, "The JCAHO Sentinel Even Policy: Concerns and Alternatives," *Health Law Digest* 26 (1998): 3–11.

39. The Federal Aviation Administration's Aviation Safety Reporting System (ASRS) uses the National Aeronautics and Space Administration as a third party to receive aviation safety reports. Reports made using this system are prohibited from use for enforcement purposes. 14 CFR sec. 91.25 (2001). There are some exceptions, as when the information involves criminal offenses or accidents outlined in paragraphs 7a(1) and 7a(2). Also, when a violation of federal aviation regulations is made known to the Federal Aviation Administration from a source other than the ASRS, appropriate action can be taken.

40. 42 U.S.C sec. 11, 101–111, 152.

41. Liang, "The Adverse Event of Unaddressed Medical Error."

42. Liang, "The Adverse Event of Unaddressed Medical Error."

43. See a measure introduced in the U.S. Senate entitled, The Patient Safety and Quality Improvement Act, (S.2590) and a companion bill introduced in the U.S. House of Representatives, The Patient Safety and Quality Improvement Act (H.R. 4889).

Chapter Two

1. F. A. Rozovsky, *Consent to Treatment: A Practical Guide,* 3rd ed. (Gaithersburg, Md.: Aspen, 2002 Suppl.). See generally Chapter One.

2. Rozovsky, *Consent to Treatment.*

3. Rozovsky, *Consent to Treatment.*

4. Rozovsky, *Consent to Treatment.*

5. Rozovsky, *Consent to Treatment.*

6. See 210 Ill. Comp. Stat. Ann. 87/a et seq. (1994).

7. "National Standards on Culturally and Linguistically Appropriate Services (CLAS) in Health Care," *Federal Register,* Dec. 22, 2000, pp. 80865 et seq.

8. Aikins v. St. Helena Hospital, 843 F. Supp. 1329 (N.D. Cal. 1994).
9. "National Standards on Culturally and Linguistically Appropriate Services (CLAS) in Health Care."
10. Rozovsky, *Consent to Treatment*. See Chapter Two, "Exceptions to the Rule."
11. Rozovsky, *Consent to Treatment*.
12. Rozovsky, *Consent to Treatment*.
13. Rozovsky, *Consent to Treatment*. See Chapter One.
14. Rozovsky, *Consent to Treatment*.
15. Rozovsky, *Consent to Treatment*. See Chapter 12.
16. Rozovsky, *Consent to Treatment*.

Chapter Seven

1. American Society for Healthcare Risk Management, *Perspective on Disclosure of Unanticipated Outcome Information* (Chicago: American Society for Healthcare Risk Management, July 2001).

INDEX

171

Consent forms: for care providers, 41–42; distinction between consent process and, 11, 18–19, 48–49, 160; formats for, 40–41

Consent process, 17–52; case examples of, 45–52; clinical benefits of, 17–20; common knowledge in, 35–36; computerized, 19; distinction between consent forms and, 11, 18–19, 48–49, 160; and family members, 31; legal ability in, 21–22; mental capability in, 22; modulating patient expectations in, 36–37; as patient safety tool, 39–40; practical issues in, 30–39; session approach to, 34; tips for facilitating, 22–23; as tool for patient communication, 18, 19–20, 32, 44–45. *See also* Consent

Consent to treatment. *See* Consent

Consumer information, health care, 8, 31, 89, 128–133

Conversations (with colleagues): about quitting medicine after death of patient, 133–136; about refusal to meet with patient and family, 97–99

Conversations (with patients/families): about anger based on misperception of events, 124–128; about care providers' disagreement over care management in front of patient, 76–84; about fetal death with patient-chosen VBAC, 118–122; about Internet information on hysterectomies, 128–133; about medical errors with no adverse consequences, 122–124; about mismanagement of care in cases of fetal death, 72–76, 84–88; about patient's correct interpretation of poorly managed case, 84–88; about relationship between obstetrician's fatigue and maternal death, 103–109; about request for legal representation in counseling session, 116–118; about slang usage by care providers, 99–103; about untreated hypertension resulting in fetal death, 89–94; care providers' apprehension about, 55–57; caution on using medical terminology in, 23, 140; discussing past loss experiences in, 147; documentation of, 59–60; over telephone or by e-mail, 142–146; religion as topic in, 148; structured approach to, 55–60; when medical record contains inconsistencies, 111–115. *See also* Appointments, postpartum; Counseling sessions; Delivering bad news

Costs, of disclosing adverse outcomes, 10

Counseling sessions: as approach to consent process, 34; furniture arrangement for, 154–156; genetic, over telephone or by e-mail, 142–146; patient requesting legal representation at, 116–118; topics for discussion in, 23–24. *See also* Appointments, postpartum

Cremation of stillborn babies, mismanagement of issue of, 64, 66, 69, 73

Cultural attitudes: toward autopsies of stillborn babies, 69–70; toward communications in obstetrics, 25–26

D

Deaths, due to medical errors, 2. *See also* Fetal death; Maternal death

Deceit, as basis of consent litigation, 43

Delivering bad news: discussing patient's past loss experiences when, 147; by e-mail, 142–146; mentioning religion when, 148; to non-English-speaking patients, 139–142; over telephone, 142–146. *See also* Conversations (with patients/families); Disclosure of adverse outcomes

Disclosure of adverse outcomes: care provider apprehension about, 55–57; and drivers for increased disclosure of health care information, 2–9; evidentiary protection for, 12–15; financial cost of, 10; insurance industry perspective on, 8–9; policy and procedure on, 161–162; practical conditions hindering, 11; research on, 9–10; risk of litigation with, 9–10; scripting, 160–161; transparent approach to, 163–164. *See also* Delivering bad news; Full disclosure

Documentation: caution on altering, 153; of consent, 40–41; of conversations, information in, 59–60, 150–151, 161; date/time on notes in, 150–151; good, characteristics of, 150–153; hospital vs. office-based, 149–150; inconsistencies in, 111–115; legibility of handwriting in, 151–152; personal opinions in, 152–153; purposes of, 148–149, 161

Doing What Counts for Patient Safety: Federal Actions to Reduce Medical Errors and Their Impact (Quality Interagency Coordination Task Force), 2

Duress, used to obtain consent, 38–39

E

E-mail, delivering bad news by, 142–146

Education, in conversations, 57

Emergencies: implied consent in, 26–27; patient/family anger over misperceived events in, 124–128

Empathy, expressed in conversations, 57

Employers, patient safety standards advocated by, 7–8

Enterprise liability theory, 3–4

Evidentiary protection, disclosure of adverse outcomes, 12–15

Evidentiary use laws, 3

Examination rooms, procedures for showing respect to patients in, 157–158

Expectations of care: modulating, 36–37; unrealistic, identifying and managing, 51–52

Expert witnesses, 44

Extended family, evaluating understanding of, 58–59

F

Facts, in conversations, 57

Family members: and consent process, 31; evaluating understanding of, 58–59; included in obstetric appointments, 25–26

Fatigue, obstetrician, in case of maternal death, 103–109

FEARED acronym for structuring conversations, 57–60

Federal Aviation Administration, Aviation Safety Reporting System (ASRS), 168n39

Federal government: and evidentiary protection for disclosure, 12–13, 14; perspective on patient communication, 2–3, 6–7

Federal Torts Claims Act, 10

Fetal death: delivering news of, to non-English-speaking patient, 139–142; mismanagement of care in cases of, 61–76, 84–88; with patient-chosen VBAC, 118–122; patient's correct interpretation of events leading to, 84–88; untreated maternal hypertension contributing to, 89–94. *See also* Stillborn babies

Fetal movement, decreased, responding to patient reports of, 62, 65, 72, 84

Fraud, as basis of consent litigation, 43

Full disclosure, 53–60; structuring conversations for, 57–60; value of, 53–55. *See also* Disclosure of adverse outcomes

Furniture arrangement, counseling sessions, 154–156

G

Gender of care providers, cultural sensitivity to, 25–26

Genetic counseling, over telephone or by e-mail, 142–146

Government Accounting Office (GAO), 5

H

Hand washing, provider, 158

Handwriting, in documentation, 151–152

Health care professionals. *See* Care providers; Obstetricians

Health Care Quality Improvement Act (HCQIA), limited protection for reporting data, 12, 13

Hearing-impaired patients, 25

History taking, 17–18, 32–33

Honesty, about medical errors with no adverse consequences, 122–124

Hospitals: consumer information on, 8; Leapfrog standards for, 7–8

Hypertension, untreated, contributing to fetal death, 89–94

Hysterectomies, Internet information on, 128–133

I

Immunizations, reporting system for adverse events following, 13
Implied consent, emergencies, 26–27
Impracticality of consent exception to rules of consent, 27–28
Information: available to consumers on Internet, 8, 31, 89, 128–133; desired by obstetric patients, 23–24; given by care provider vs. received by patient, 136–138; material or significant, 33–34; methods of supplying, 30–31
Informed consent. *See* Consent; Consent process
Institute of Medicine (IOM), 2, 3
Insurance industry, perspective on disclosure of adverse outcomes, 8–9
Internet, patient information on, 8, 31, 89, 128–133
Interpreters, 19–20, 25, 139–142

J

Joint Commission on Accreditation of Healthcare Organizations (JCAHO): accreditation by, 4–5; hospital performance data published by, 8; patient involvement encouraged by, 6; patient safety standards, 5–6; signed consent documents encouraged by, 48

L

Language issues: forms of address for patients, 158; medical terminology, 23, 140; slang, 99–103; using interpreters, 19–20, 25, 139–142
Lawsuits. *See* Litigation
Lawyer, patient requesting presence of, at counseling session, 116–118
"Leapfrog Group," proposed patient safety standards, 7–8
Legal ability, consent process, 21–22
Legal action. *See* Litigation
Liability: and apologies, 164; enterprise liability theory, 3–4; for lack of informed consent, 43–44
Licensure of health professionals, 3

Lifestyle issues, management of, in consent process, 46–48
Limited-English-speaking patients, using interpreters with, 19–20, 25, 139–142
Litigation: apprehension about potential for, 56–57; for lack of informed consent, 27, 28, 43–44; lessening chances of, 159; risk of, with disclosure of medical errors, 9–10
Loss, discussing patient's past experiences of, 147

M

Making Health Care Safer: A Critical Analysis of Patient Safety Practices (UCSF-Standard Evidence-Based Practice Center), 2
Management of care: care providers' disagreement on, in front of patient, 76–84; contributing to death of fetus, patient interpretation of, 84–88; with fetal death, 61–76, 84–88; poor, patient correctly interpreting, 84–88
Manufacturer and User Facility Device Experience Database, 13
Material information, 33–34
Maternal death: care provider considering quitting medicine after, 133–136; fatigue of obstetrician in case of, 103–109
Medicaid Patients Rights Standards, 2
Medical devices, reporting system for adverse events with use of, 13
Medical errors: consumer information on, 8; deaths per year due to, 2; disclosure of, and litigation, 9–10; with no adverse consequences, 122–124. *See also* Adverse event reporting systems
Medical records. *See* Documentation
Medical terminology, caution on using, 23, 140
Mental capability, consent process, 22
Misrepresentation, as basis of consent litigation, 43
Mistakes. *See* Medical errors

Questions: "drill-down" approach to, 33, 39; from patient, 23, 31

R

"Refusal to be informed" cases, 29–30

Relating back: to check patient understanding, 34–35, 58; communication given vs. received revealed by, 136–138; in consent process, 34–35

Religion, as topic in conversations, 148

Reservation of rights letter, 9

Revocation of consent, 37–38

Risk factors: consent as tool for managing, 39–40; revealed in history taking, 17–18

S

Session approach to consent process, 34

Significant information, 33–34

Slang, bad outcome's significance minimized by, 99–103

"Speak Up: Help Prevent Errors in Your Care" (JCAHO), 6

Special Nutritional Adverse Event Monitoring System, 13

Spouses: consent process involving, 31; as intermediary in communication with patient, 26

Standard of care, and consent litigation, 43–44

Standard of disclosure, and consent litigation, 44

State governments: evidentiary protection for disclosure, 13; laws on interpreter services, 25; patient safety standards, 7–8; perspective on patient communication, 3–4

Stillborn babies: autopsies of, 63–64, 66, 68, 73; cremation of, 64, 66, 69, 73; family time with, 63, 66, 68, 70, 74; parental requests for care of, 64, 70, 74; photographs of, 63, 66, 68, 73. *See also* Fetal death

T

Telephone, delivering bad news over, 142–146

Ten-minute chat, 157

Therapeutic privilege exception to rules of consent, 28

Time issues: allowing family time with stillborn baby, 63, 66, 68, 70, 74; date/time notation on documentation entries, 150–151; giving patient time to absorb information, 22–23, 62–63, 66, 67, 72; impatient patients, 50–52; session approach to consent process, 34; ten-minute chat, 157; timing of first postpartum appointment after fetal death, 67, 70–71, 74

To Err Is Human: Building a Safer Health System (Institute of Medicine), 2, 3, 5

Transportation, after receiving news of fetal death, 63, 66, 67, 73

U

Unanticipated outcomes, and JCAHO, 5–6. *See also* Disclosure of adverse outcomes

Understanding: of extended family, 58–59; of patient, 34–35, 58, 136–138

University of California at San Francisco (UCSF), Standard Evidence-Based Practice Center, 2

U.S. Department of Health and Human Services: Office of Civil Rights, 25; Office of the Inspector General (OIG), 5

U.S. Food and Drug Administration (FDA), 2; adverse event reporting systems, 12–13

V

Vaccine Adverse Event Reporting System, 12–13

Vaginal birth after cesarean section (VBAC), fetal death with, 118–122

Veterans Administration (VA) Medical Center (Lexington, KY), cost benefit of disclosure policy of, 10

W

Ward rounds, effective provider-patient communication on, 156–157

Writing, in documentation, 151–152

Printed in the United States
75728LV00004B/4-24

9 780787 966546